Pulmonary Physiology for Clinicians

Marc Lavietes • Andrew Berman

Pulmonary Physiology for Clinicians

A Focused Guide

Springer

Marc Lavietes
Medicine (Pulmonary and Critical Care)
Rutgers, New Jersey Medical School
Newark, NJ, USA

Andrew Berman
Medicine (Pulmonary and Critical Care)
Rutgers, New Jersey Medical School
Newark, NJ, USA

ISBN 978-3-032-24302-7 ISBN 978-3-032-24303-4 (eBook)
https://doi.org/10.1007/978-3-032-24303-4

This Springer imprint is published by the registered company Springer Nature Switzerland AG
The registered company address is: Gewerbestrasse 11, 6330 Cham, Switzerland

This book is dedicated to my mentor, Dr. Dudley F. Rochester who was intensely devoted both to the study of pulmonary physiology and to its clinical teaching. His empathy, sincerity, and humility were unique among his peers.

Marc Lavietes, MD

I dedicate this book to my students, whose inquisitiveness renews my passion for pulmonary physiology.

Andrew Berman, MD

Preface

Pulmonary function testing is an important component of several determinations used to evaluate respiratory health. Others include history, physical examination, serological and skin testing, and imaging studies. Clinicians and epidemiologists rely on pulmonary function testing both to confirm diagnoses and to evaluate the functional status of patients and study subjects. Medical and graduate school programs offer comprehensive sections on pulmonary physiology early in their curricula as do basic physiology textbooks. Later, clinical courses and texts describe the pathophysiology of lung diseases. Their descriptions include the pulmonary function test results associated with each clinical condition. However, they offer little or no accompanying discussion of the physiological principles underlying those results. Therefore, many students do not grasp the relationships between basic physiology and the clinical application of their test results. Given a lack of understanding of underlying physiological principles, physicians often miss some of the clinical implications available to them from the interpretation of these results. It seems that while students readily understand the function of other organs, the understanding of lung physiology is sometimes enigmatic.

The goal of this book is: to integrate the interpretation of pulmonary function test results with both their physiological basis and their clinical implications. This book picks and chooses those basic concepts that are necessary to understand and interpret clinical lung function test results. To this end, many fundamental physiological concepts presented in other texts are omitted here. For one clear example: the description of the physicochemistry of hemoglobin. Basic texts all present graphs showing three variables: oxygen tension (*x*-axis), hemoglobin saturation (*y*-axis), and a third variable, either pH or temperature, represented as a continuous line or curve on the graph. This information is critical for the understanding of how oxygen first affixes to hemoglobin in the lung and is later released for uptake by the tissues. It is however not helpful for the interpretation of pulmonary function tests. On the other hand, material not found elsewhere is presented here because of its importance for the interpretation of test results. For example, we describe at length the protocols for the performance of each test. Knowledge of these protocols and procedures is important for both the technician performing the test and the clinician interpreting them. The technician, in order to achieve successful technician-patient coordination, must understand the principles governing the instructions given to the test subject. The clinician must also be familiar with test procedures. For example, when interpreting the data describing lung volume, the clinician must know that a gas dilution technique may underestimate the true lung volume of an emphysematous patent whereas plethysmography will provide more accurate data.

There are four components of a standard pulmonary function testing session. Each of the first four chapters here is devoted to one component. These include: one, evaluation of the static properties of the respiratory system; two, its dynamic properties; three, the propensity for gas to diffuse across the alveolar-pulmonary capillary membrane; and lastly the properties of the lung allowing for the matching of ventilation with perfusion (V/Q). The property of V/Q matching is quantified with surrogate measures: arterial blood gas determination in some laboratories; less invasive procedures such as measurements of oxygen saturation and end tidal pCO_2 in others. This book is then presented in sections corresponding to the laboratory protocol for lung function testing. Each section will follow the identical format: a brief commentary on the origin and evolution of the test to be described along with a detailed account of how the test is performed and the results interpreted. This is followed by comments on the clinical implications of test results and finally a review of the physiological principles governing the interpretation of each test.

Newark, NJ, USA Marc Lavietes

Contents

1 **Static Lung Volumes: The Restrictive Ventilatory Defect** 1

2 **Dynamic Lung Function: The Obstructive Ventilatory Defect** 17

3 **Diffusion** 35

4 **Matching of Ventilation (V/Q) with Perfusion: Arterial Blood Gas (ABG) Analysis** 41

5 **Respiratory Regulation** 53

6 **Exercise Testing as a Diagnostic Tool** 59

7 **Respiratory Muscle Testing** 73

Correction to: Exercise Testing as a Diagnostic Tool C1

Index 85

Static Lung Volumes: The Restrictive Ventilatory Defect

1

Clinical pulmonary function test reports usually begin with the measurements of lung volume. The notion that a lung volume, the so-called vital capacity (VC), could be measured and that the measurement could be useful to the clinician was introduced by the British physician John Hutchinson in 1846 [1]. With the spirometer he designed, Hutchinson collected and measured his subjects' exhaled air volume starting from full inflation and ending with complete deflation. He compared VC measurements from normal volunteers to those from subjects with various diseases of the respiratory system. Spirometry could not measure total lung capacity (TLC), of course, because residual volume (RV), that is, the gas remaining in the lung following full voluntary deflation, could not be expelled into the spirometer. Scientists first attempted to measure lung volumes with a hydrogen gas dilution method as long as 200 years ago. However, TLC was not measured in clinical practice until the years following World War Two (WW2) when new technology made the measurement of RV and thus TLC more practical. Helium (He) and nitrogen (N2) meters enabled measurement of RV by either gas equilibration or washout maneuvers [2]. The notion that FRC (functional residual capacity, or the volume of gas remaining in the lung following a tidal breath) could be measured by a gas compression method during a panting maneuver was proposed late in the nineteenth century. FRC measurement would then allow computation of RV,

M. Lavietes, A. Berman, *Pulmonary Physiology for Clinicians*,
https://doi.org/10.1007/978-3-032-24303-4_1

because a portion of FRC (called expiratory reserve volume or ERV) could be collected in the spirometer and thus RV could be calculated. Precise plethysmographic measurements were not possible until after WW2, however, when pressure transducers capable of recording the small pressure changes developed during the panting maneuver became available [3]. These laboratory methods have been confirmed by radiologic methods, first using posteroanterior and lateral chest films and more recently by computed tomography. Roentgenographic methods however are not practical for use in a clinical service lung function laboratory. Today, while the majority of clinical laboratories use the N2 washout method for their lung volume measurements, many still use either plethysmography or gas equilibration methods. It is useful for the pulmonary function test reader to be aware of the technical differences between methods. Under some clinical circumstances, the various methods may not yield exactly identical results.

A spirometry trace of the slow VC maneuver appears in Fig. 1.1. The subject, seated and wearing a nose clip, breathes through a mouthpiece. After a few tidal breaths are recorded, the subject exhales fully. He then inhales fully to TLC. Lastly, he relaxes. A few tidal breaths following the maneuver are then recorded. Exhalation before inhalation to TLC is the preferred method. This minimizes the possibility of any air trapping as the subject approaches RV. The point on the tracing at the end of each tidal breath is FRC, the thoracic gas volume at the end of each tidal breath. The technician repeats the maneuver until two maximal and reproducible takings are obtained. The reader cannot quantify FRC from this trace because the RV measurement is not available. Important measures seen here are the VC, the inspiratory capacity (IC), that is, the air volume inhaled from FRC, and the expiratory reserve volume (ERV), that is, the gas volume exhaled from FRC to RV.

RV and therefore TLC cannot be measured directly. One method often used to obtain both measurements is the multiple breath nitrogen washout method (N2 w/o). The washout provides an FRC value. Subtraction of ERV obtained from spirometry yields RV. RV + VC also obtained from spirometry yields TLC.

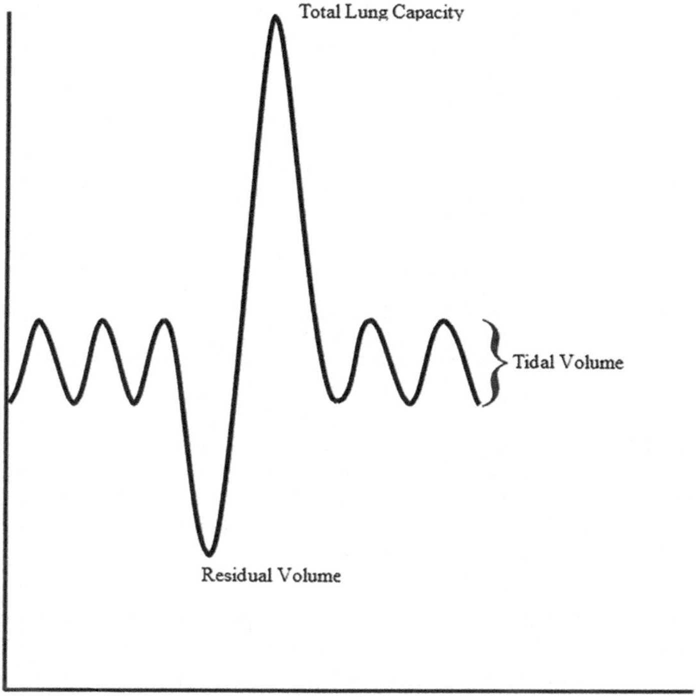

Fig. 1.1 The slow vital capacity (VC) maneuver. Vertical axis = volume. TLC – RV = VC. Functional residual capacity (FRC) is represented by the point at the end of each tidal breath. Inspiratory capacity (IC) = TLC – FRC. Expiratory reserve volume (ERV) = FRC – RV

To perform the test, the subject breathes quietly through a mouthpiece and one-way valve. At the end of a breath, that is, when the volume of gas in the lung is FRC, the technician switches the valve such that the subject now inhales 100% oxygen. All of the subject's subsequent breath is collected. Exhaled nitrogen is measured breath by breath as it is diluted and [N2] diminishes with each breath. A trace of exhaled N2 over time in a normal subject during the maneuver appears in Fig. 1.2. The process ends when expired [N2] reaches a nadir of 2%. Since [N2] in the lung is 80%, FRC is (total exhaled N2)/0.8. Conceivably the test will

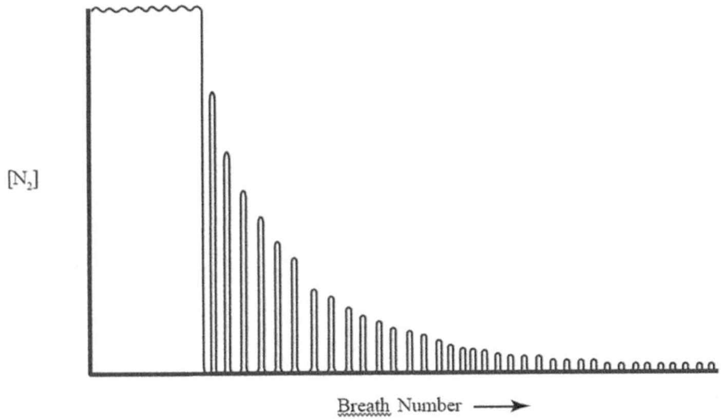

Fig. 1.2 The multiple breath nitrogen washout. Vertical axis = [N2]. Horizontal axis = sequential tidal breaths. The volume of nitrogen collected from this maneuver is used to calculate functional residual capacity. The length of time to empty the lung of nitrogen—expressed as the lung clearance index (LCI)—is a measure of airway function

overestimate FRC because nitrogen escaping from body tissues adds to the exhaled gas. The amount of nitrogen released from tissue is proportional to body weight. Tables are available that estimate nitrogen loss from tissue over time based upon body weight. These nitrogen losses are negligible however. Most protocols overlook them. The washout procedure is completed within 2–3 minutes for normal subjects. In patients with airway obstruction, however, the washout is prolonged and may require more than 10 min. Of interest here, the lung clearance index (LCI) is the total gas volume exhaled during the washout divided by FRC. It is sometimes used by pediatricians to identify subtle degrees of airway dysfunction in small children. This test is suitable for small children because it can be accomplished with a facemark rather than a mouthpiece. The term "LCI" appears often in the pediatric pulmonary literature.

A second common gas dilution method utilizes an inert tracer, often helium, to measure FRC volume. In this procedure, the subject, seated, breathes quietly via a mouthpiece and valve. The tidal breath is monitored. At the end of a breath, the valve is turned so that the subject is now rebreathing from a closed system in which the initial gas volume and helium concentration (C1;V1) are known. Oxygen is added and CO2 constantly scrubbed from the system so that the end expiratory system volume is maintained constant. When equilibrium is reached, the observed helium concentration (C2) is recorded. To compute FRC, V2 – V1 + FRC. The equation then reads:

$$(\mathrm{C1})(\mathrm{V1}) = \mathrm{C2}(\mathrm{V1} + FRC)$$

Note: later in the laboratory protocol during the determination of the diffusion capacity (see below), lung volume will again be measured with an inert gas equilibration method. This is done because the diffusion capacity (DlCO) represents the product of TLC and a rate constant describing gas diffusion across the alveolar-capillary membrane. TLC and the rate constant are obtained simultaneously. In that procedure, the subject inhales inspired gas with a known concentration of an inert marker that will distribute throughout the lung (C1) along with a known concentration of carbon monoxide (CO) from RV to TLC. At the end of a 10-second breath hold, gas is rapidly exhaled. The resultant inert marker concentration (C2) is used to compute TLC:

$$TLC = (\text{Inhaled volume}) \times (\mathrm{C1}/\mathrm{C2})$$

This procedure provides a reliable estimate of TLC in normal subjects or those with small lung volumes. The 10-s breath hold is often inadequate for complete equilibrium of the marker via pendelluft ventilation in patients with airway obstruction, however. This method often underestimates TLC in those subjects. The multiple breath equilibration of helium approximates TLC well in most patients. It may underestimate TLC in a few patients with diffuse emphysema or large poorly communicating bullae, however.

Plethysmography determines FRC by a method involving gas compression. The subject is seated in an airtight chamber or box called a plethysmograph while breathing through a manually operated valve. The subject is coached to begin panting at the end of a tidal breath, that is, when the volume of thoracic gas is FRC.

The operator closes the shutter for a few seconds. The subject continues to pant, thus alternately compressing and expanding the thoracic gas. Simultaneous measurements of chamber and airway pressures made during this maneuver allow for computation of the compressed gas, that is, FRC.

The process uses the equation: (V1) (P1) = (V2) (P2), where V1 = FRC and P1 = atmospheric pressure. An infinite number of V2s and P2s are developed during the panting procedure with smaller V2 produced during the expiratory phase of panting, larger V2s during the inspiratory cycle. Since these changes are very small, the equation is rewritten as follows:

$$(\mathrm{P1})(\mathrm{V1}) = (\mathrm{P1} + dP)(\mathrm{V1} + dP): \text{where d} = \text{delta, or change}$$

dP is measured directly from the mouthpiece. dV is measured indirectly. It is assumed that during the expiratory cycle of panting, the thoracic gas, FRC, is compressed while the gas volume with the plethysmograph expands. That volume can be calculated from the decrease in box pressure measured from the pressure transducer. The reverse is true during the inspiratory panting cycle. These volume changes are equal and opposite. They create a cyclic change in pressure within the enclosed space of the plethysmograph. That pressure can be calibrated so as to correspond to a volume change. Thus, V2 is obtained from the cyclic pressure change within the plethysmograph. The equation rearranges to:

$$FRC = (\mathrm{P\,barometric} - 47)(dP\,\mathrm{box}) / dP\,\mathrm{mouth}),$$

where 47 = water vapor pressure.

The slope can be read directly as the slope seen on x-y recording of the oscillating pressures as seen on an oscilloscope during the panting maneuver. Note that gas distal to poorly communicating areas of lung or gas within poorly communicating bullae are reliably measured by gas compression. Thus in patients with obstructive lung physiology, plethysmographic measures of FRC and TLC are more likely than measures with gas dilution methods to yield TLC measurements equal to those obtained from an X-ray or computed tomography exam [4]. Conversely, the panting maneuver may slightly overestimate volume in COPD patients because pressure may not fully equilibrate between alveoli and mouthpiece during panting in those patients [5].

Conventionally, clinicians report values for TLC and its subdivisions as percentage of a predicted value [6]. Adjustments are made for age, sex, and height. If one computes an average TLC volume for a group of healthy 20-year-old women 66″ in height, for example, two standard deviations from the mean will correspond roughly to a range from 80% to 120% of the mean value. Thus convention holds that 80% of a predicted value is the lower limit of normal for all static lung volume measurements. There is some current literature recommending the use of z-scores rather than the language of percentage predicted. In practice, however, z-scores are not widely used. Schemes for grading functional impairment differ from laboratory to laboratory. One common grading scheme is as follows:

Mild restrictive defect: 70%–80% predicted
Moderate: 60%–69% predicted
Severe: 35%–49% predicted
Very severe: <35% predicted

Traditionally adjustments in predicted values have been made for race. The notion has been: Black persons have lower predicted values than Caucasian people because genetically, trunk/body height ratios differ for racial groups. This notion has been challenged recently and race correction is now discouraged. Epidemiologists recognize that lung volume differences may reflect acquired rather than genetic factors given that nutrition, prenatal healthcare, and many other factors differ between races. Authors also have pointed out that the use of race correction may be detrimental to the health outcomes of Black people [7]. Use of a race-specific grading scheme will categorize some Black subjects who with a universal grading system would be classified as mild restrictive defect as having normal lungs. Those subjects may then be denied surveillance or other preventative care measures that are intended only for those with minimal impairment.

Finally, it should be apparent to the clinician that the difference between 79% and 80% predicted is negligible.

The clinician or test reader must determine that each given test has been executed correctly and that the data are true. This process of quality assurance is achieved primarily by critical analysis of the timed forced vital capacity (FVC) curve, to be discussed later. The reader, however, may assess the quality of the TLC determination by comparing the measured TLC to the TLC determined later (referred to as VA) during the diffusion capacity test. TLC and VA should be identical. Since VA is determined by the equilibration of a label during a 10-s breath hold, equilibration may be insufficient in COPD subjects. Therefore, in some COPD patients, VA may underestimate TLC. Test results showing VA to be far greater than TLC reflect laboratory or patient performance error.

One final caveat. How does the reader interpret volume when the VC is diminished and the TLC normal? Often, a subject performs only the FVC in a screening test session. In this case, the FVC is the only volume measurement available for analysis. The reader must make his judgment on lung volume based upon the FVC alone. On occasion, in the course of a complete study, the VC may be minimally reduced while the TLC is normal. To illustrate, let us consider a few clinical situations. First, consider a patient with a low (L5 -S1) spinal cord injury with an otherwise normal lung. VC will be diminished and RV elevated because expiratory muscles function poorly. Since inspiratory muscles are intact, TLC is normal. A second example is the emphysema patient whose RV is elevated because of airway closure but TLC is again normal or minimally increased while VC is diminished. Patients with these disparate clinical conditions have similar static functions. One has normal lung. The other, emphysematous lung. The take-home message is: test results are best interpreted in conjunction with clinical information.

Differential dx of Restrictive Defect

Patients with a restrictive ventilatory defect fall into three broad diagnostic categories: those having diseases involving the lung parenchyma, the chest wall, and the neuromuscular systems. The term "chest wall" used here broadly refers to all structures that participate in cyclic respiratory motion outside of the lung, for example, spinal column and rib cage, intercostal muscles, diaphragm, and abdominal wall. While a diminished TLC defines a restrictive defect, there are many different combinations and permutations of the volume subdivisions, each depending on the underlying pathology of the respiratory system.

Disease processes characterized by either fibrosis, cellular infiltration, or edema of the lung parenchyma produce a restrictive ventilatory defect. These conditions prevent full expansion of the lung. They produce a similar pattern of lung function. Inflation to high lung volumes, for example, IC, is impaired. Lower lung volumes, for example, RV, are less affected. Thus the expected pattern is TLC, VC, IC, and FRC are reduced to a greater degree than RV. The RV/TLC ratio is increased. This pattern is also seen in processes involving alveolar filling, for example, pneumonia, as well as large airway obstruction with resultant collapse of a lobar segment. Lung restriction in atelectasis may be minimal, however, because collapse of one segment or lobe may accompanied by compensatory expansion of the remaining lung.

There is no one profile to describe the alterations in the subdivisions of lung volume that fits all patients with chest wall disorders. In particular, RV may be diminished, normal, or elevated depending upon the functional characteristics of the chest wall in each given condition. In obesity, for example, RV and FRC are diminished. IC may be normal, but the sum of IC + FRC is always reduced. Contrast this with the somewhat rare condition ankylosing spondylitis in which the chest wall is rigid but fixed at a volume slightly greater than that of the normal chest wall. Thus, in this condition RV—and sometimes FRC as well—is elevated while TLC is reduced. Conditions in which abdominal pressure is elevated such as ascites, pregnancy, and/or gastric distension also

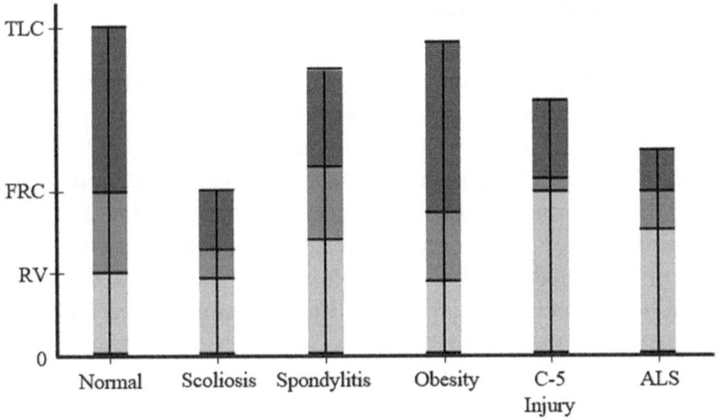

Fig. 1.3 Total lung capacity and its subdivisions in various disorders of the thoracic cage. Hatched lines represent TLC, FRC, and RV, respectively. Note that each condition has its own specific pattern of IC + ERV + RV. Each pattern is a function of the unique properties of the chest wall in each given condition as represented by its volume-pressure characteristic on its Fenn-Rahn diagram (Redrawn from Ref. [9])

reduce TLC [8]. In these cases, ERV and thus FRC are diminished while IC is normal. TlLC is minimally reduced.

Normal FRC is characteristic of lung function in patients with myopathy. Given global muscle weakness, both IV and ERV are decreased while RV is elevated.

Each disorder of the chest wall may be characterized by its own unique configuration of TLC and its subdivisions. These are illustrated in Fig. 1.3 [9].

Physiology

The mechanical properties of the normal respiratory system are described by the classic volume/pressure (V/P) diagram of Rahn et al. [10]. They are shown in Fig. 1.4. Look first at the V/P characteristic of a normal lung. Where the inflation curve flattens at TLC, the corresponding pressure is 30 cm H20. This pressure is the lung recoil pressure at TLC for animals throughout the animal

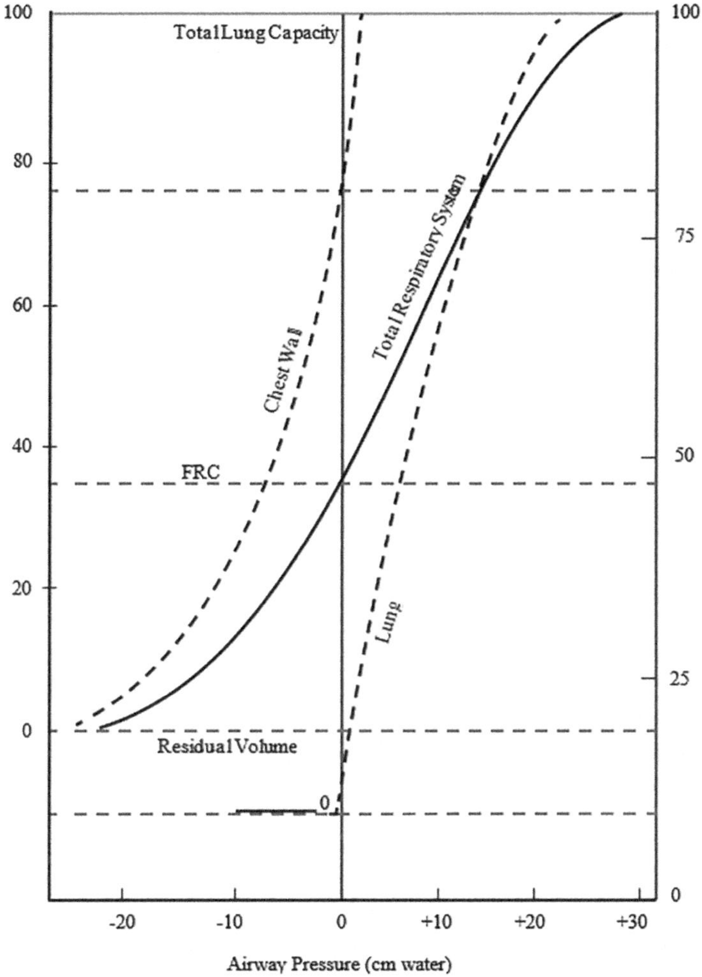

Fig. 1.4 The classic V/P Fenn-Rahn diagram with volume versus pressure curves for the chest wall, total respiratory system, and lung is shown from left to right. Note that at low and mid lung volumes, the resting position of the chest wall is reached by expansion, not retraction

kingdom, from mouse to elephant. Note that the entire inflation curve lies on the positive side of zero, that is, a lung inflated to any given volume will collapse. This is apparent to anyone who has observed a thoracic surgery procedure. If the chest is opened without pressure being applied via an ET tube, the lung collapses. Look next at the curve for the normal chest wall. Until the lung reaches approximately 70% of TLC, the curve lies on the negative side of zero, that is, the chest wall tends to expand at lower volumes. As the thoracic surgeon opens the chest cavity, the rib cage appears to expand slightly. This would be predicted by the V/P diagram. Finally, look at the respiratory system curve, that is, the summation of lung and chest wall pressures and volumes. When one reads an airway pressure from a ventilator monitor, for example, that summation pressure represents this pressure, the summation of chest wall and lung recoil.

Note that at FRC, the pressures are equal and opposite. Thus for normals and most patients, FRC represents a resting position. For this reason, the laboratory technician initiates helium dilution or nitrogen washout procedures at the end of a tidal breath. Note that there is one exception to this truth: positive end expiratory pressure (PEEP). Extrinsic PEEP, or pressure applied to the airway via an ET tube at end expiration, is obvious. Intrinsic PEEP, observed in patients with severe airway obstruction, occurs when the subject fails to exhale to the resting position before initiating his next breath.

The volume/pressure curve of a patient with interstitial pulmonary fibrosis superimposed upon the normal V/P diagram appears in Fig. 1.5. Note that in order for FRC to represent a resting position, FRC must decrease so that lung and chest wall recoil remain equal and opposite. Similarly, the curve depicting the abnormal chest wall characteristic of an obese subject also superimposed upon normal appears in Fig. 1.6. Finally, the changes in the V/P characteristic of the chest wall with abdominal distension require comment. An experiment in which abdominal distention was induced experimentally by the installation of 1.0 L of water into the stomachs of volunteer subjects showed acute change in gastric volume is accompanied by equivalent changes in intrathoracic and intra-abdominal pressures [11]. These changes in rib cage and

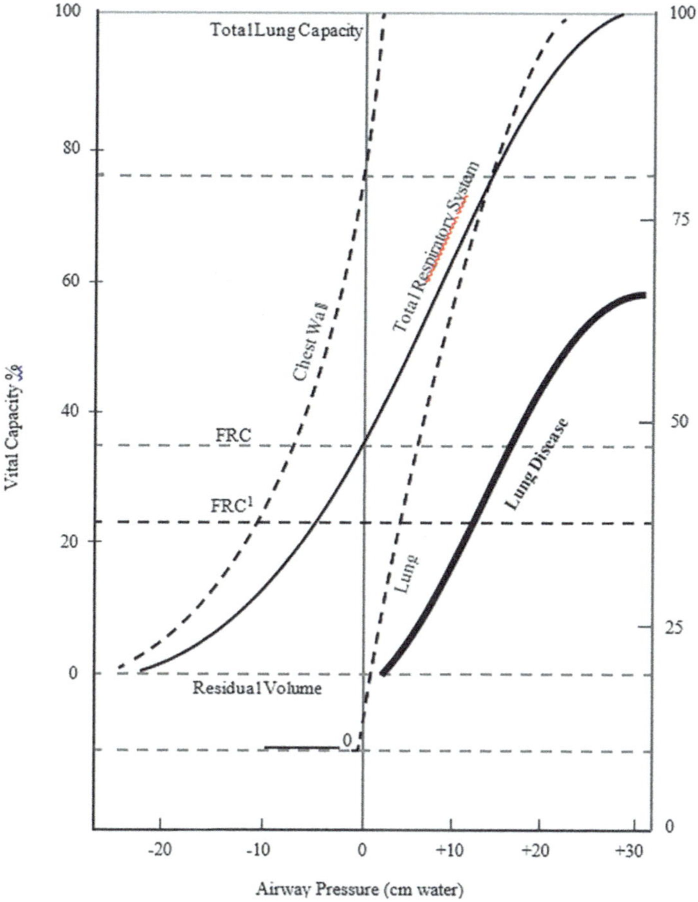

Fig. 1.5 The V/P characteristic of the lung in a patient with diffuse disease of the lung parenchyma superimposed upon the normal Fenn-Rahn V/P diagram. FRC prime = FRC for the patient with diffuse lung disease. Note that because of the increased lung recoil, resting FRC is diminished

abdominal shape and volume may differ, however, presumably because the compliances of the two compartments differ. Volume change is distributed between rib cage expansion, abdominal wall expansion, and a decrease in end expiratory lung volume. This is

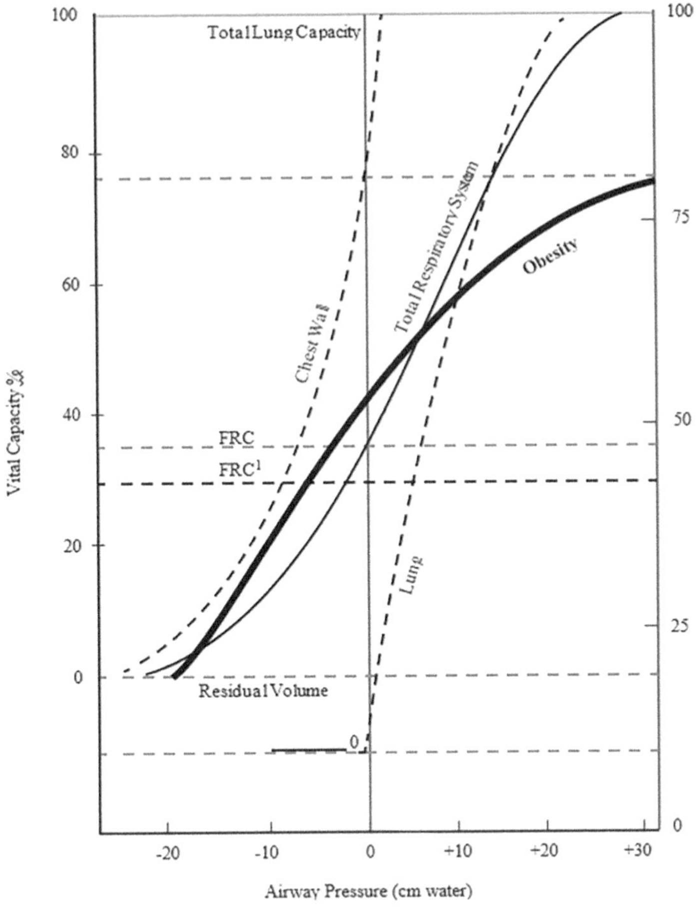

Fig. 1.6 The V/P characteristic of the chest wall in an obese subject superimposed upon normal. FRC prime = FRC for the obese patient. Note that because of the diminished outward recoil of the chest wall, resting FRC is diminished

so because at the end of a breath, the diaphragm is dome shaped with its outer edges apposed to the rib cage. Thus with increases of intra-abdominal pressure, the lower rib cage is expanded by that same pressure acting upon the lower rib cage. Note that with hyperinflation, the diaphragm of the emphysema patient is flattened at rest or early in inspiration. This reduces the efficiency of the diaphragm and contributes to the dyspnea the patient experiences. The effects of obesity or cirrhosis with minimal ascites upon static lung volumes would be expected to differ from that of ascites because their effect upon the distensibility of the abdominal wall would differ from that of ascites.

Measurements of Respiratory System Recoil Pressure in the Intensive Care Setting

Airway pressure recorded from within the endotracheal tube is continuously monitored in intubated patients. With the airway briefly occluded at end inspiration, the so-called plateau pressure recorded in the absence of airflow represents the static respiratory system recoil pressure. Since the chest wall is compliant at or around FRC, increases in this recoil pressure invariably reflect pathologic changes within the lung parenchyma. When positive end expiratory pressure (PEEP) is instituted, the difference between the plateau pressure and the end expiratory pressure (PEEP) is referred to as the driving pressure. Measurement of driving pressure provides prognostic information and guides in decision-making regarding tidal volume settings in heavily sedated patients. One analysis of data pooled from nine published trials showed strong inverse correlation between driving pressure and mortality, more so than with either pressure alone [12]. This supports the notion that cyclical stretch rather than sustained stretch is most harmful to the lung.

References

1. Petty TL. John Hutchinson's mysterious machine revisited. Chest. 2002;121(5):219S–23S.
2. Brown R, Leith DE, Enright PL. Multiple breath helium dilution measurement of lung volumes in adults. Eur Respir J. 1998;11:246–55.

3. DuBois AB, Botelho SY, Bedell GN, Marshall R, Comroe JH Jr. A rapid plethysmographic method for measuring thoracic gas volume: a comparison with a nitrogen washout method for measuring functional residual capacity in normal subjects. J Clin Invest. 1956;35:322–6.
4. Brugman TM, Morris JF, Temple WP. Comparison of lung volume measurements by single breath helium and multiple breath nitrogen equilibration methods in normal subjects and COPD patients. Respiration. 1986;49:52–60.
5. Sue DY. Measurements of lung volumes in patients with obstructive lung disease. Ann Am Thoracic Soc. 2013;10(5):525–30.
6. Stanojevic S, Wade A, Stocks J. Reference values for lung function: past, present and future. Eur Respir J. 2010;36:12–9.
7. Vyas DA, Eisenstein LG, Jones DS. The race-correction debates—progress, tensions and future directions. N Engl J Med. 2025;393(10):1029–36.
8. Hanson RA, Ritter AB, Duran W, Lavietes MH. Ascites: its effect upon static inflation of the respiratory system. Am Rev Respir Dis. 1990;142:39–42.
9. Bergofsky EH. Respiratory failure in disorders of the thoracic cage. Am Rev Respir Dis. 1979;119:643–69.
10. Rahn H, Otis AB, Chadwick LE, Fenn WO. The pressure volume diagram of the thorax and lung. Am J Physiol. 1946;2:161.
11. Gilroy RJ, Lavietes MH, Loring SH, Mangura BT, Mead J. Respiratory mechanical effects of abdominal distension. J Appl Physiol. 1985;58:1997–2003.
12. Amato MBP, Meade MO, Slutsky AS, Brochard L, Costa ELV, Schoenfeld DA, et al. Driving pressure and survival in the acute respiratory distress syndrome. N Engl J Med. 2015;372(8):747–55.

Dynamic Lung Function: The Obstructive Ventilatory Defect

2

Spirometry

The spirometer was introduced by John Hutchinson in mid-1800's to measure the volume of air in the lungs, which he termed "vital capacity." Over the next 100 years, this device evolved from a quantification of a static lung volume to one that also measures dynamic airflow, with the notable additions of the forced expiratory volume in one second (FEV1) and the "timed vital capacity" (which was the forerunner to the FEV1/FVC ratio) [1]. With contemporary digital recording equipment, the continuous measure of the slope of the FVC curve can now be measured and data can be presented in either a volume-time or a flow-volume format. Today the spirometer is a widely used tool to diagnose airway disease and monitor parenchymal lung diseases.

Anatomy and Physiology

An obstructive ventilatory defect occurs when the flow of air is diminished because of increased airway resistance. The pathology is characterized by airway narrowing. Airway narrowing can take place in the upper or extra thoracic airways (from the nasal cavity to the larynx) or the lower or intrathoracic airways (from the trachea to the respiratory bronchioles). Flow limitation is most pro-

M. Lavietes, A. Berman, *Pulmonary Physiology for Clinicians*,
https://doi.org/10.1007/978-3-032-24303-4_2

nounced in the upper or proximal intrathoracic airways, those airways having an internal diameter greater than 2 mm. Specifically, those airways have cartilaginous support [2]. These airways serve to conduct inspired air to the distal gas exchanging regions of the lung [3]. Air flows through a series of branching tubes which progressively increase in number as they divide. The small airways begin from approximately the eighth generation of branching and extend to the respiratory bronchioles [2]. These small airways do not contain cartilage, but rather are supported by surrounding alveoli. Under normal circumstances, the alveoli do not collapse because of their surfactant-like lining that lowers surface tension (applying the Law of LaPlace). Through radial attachments, the open alveoli exert a tethering effect on the small airways which increases with inspiration and decreases with expiration. In emphysema, the tethering effect on the small airway is lost because of the destruction of radial attachments between the small airways and surrounding alveoli. This leads to a loss of support that allows the airways to narrow and collapse during exhalation. This elevates airway resistance and causes airflow limitation and air trapping. The concepts of the equal pressure point and dynamic airway compression will be discussed later.

Another important difference between large and small intrathoracic airways is their cross-sectional area which increases exponentially in the small airways where there are numerous parallel paths [3]. While the resistance of a tube is inversely proportional to the fourth power of its radius (Poiseuille's Law), the large number of small airways are arranged in parallel, and thus dramatically reduce the overall resistance as these airways essentially function as a collective pathway. Thus, resistance here is lower than the larger upper airways. As the velocity of a gas is flow divided by cross-sectional area, air travels much more slowly in the small airways. Note: airflow also diminishes in all airways during normal sleep. Obstructive sleep apnea is the condition manifested by snoring if the extrathoracic airways collapse and inspiratory flow ceases entirely. This chapter will concentrate solely on expiratory flow limitation in the intrathoracic airways. Clinically, expiratory flow limitation occurs in diseases such as asthma, emphysema, and bronchiectasis. Patients present with symptoms including cough, wheezing, and shortness of breath, depending on the degree airflow reduction.

The intrathoracic airways are divided into the large (proximal) and small (distal) airways. The large airways begin with the trachea and end at the level of the subsegmental bronchi. These airways enable air to reach the alveoli where gas exchange will take place. In a healthy lung, the small airways contribute only about 10% of the total resistance to flow because they are so numerous [2]. In patients with COPD, the small airways become the primary site of obstruction. Their contribution to total resistance increases substantially. Early changes may not be detectable by routine spirometry measurements, however. Hence, the label for this area is the "silent zone" [4].

Dynamic lung volume over time is quantified by routine spirometry. In this procedure, the subject makes a maximal forced exhalation followed by inhalation into a flowmeter. A nose clip in place ensures that all air is exhaled through the mouthpiece, thus producing valid reproducible data: the FEV1, FVC, and the flow volume loop (see Fig. 2.1). The procedure starts with inspiration to TLC, followed by an immediate forceful expiration, a maneuver which must be sustained with coaching until the patient can no longer exhale. This is followed by maximal inspiration back to TLC. While vital capacity can be measured both during inha-

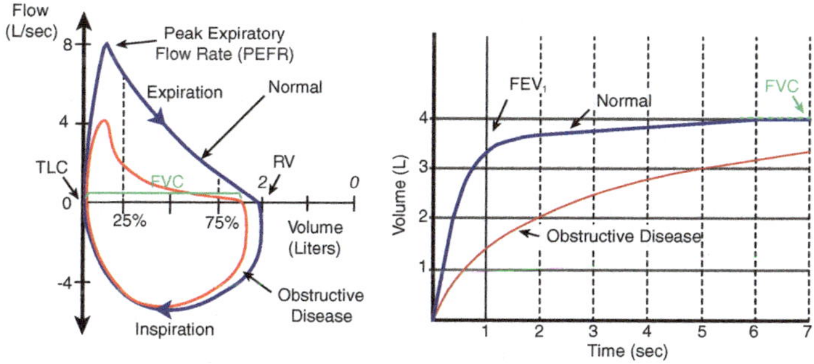

Fig. 2.1 Flow-volume loop and volume-time plot. Blue represents an individual with normal lungs; red, an individual with airway obstruction

lation (IVC) and exhalation (FVC), only the exhalation portion is standardized, in terms of reproducibility and reference values. In the healthy individual, however, IVC and FVC should be comparable. In patients with significant airway obstruction, on the other hand, IVC tends to be greater than FVC. This difference increases as the degree of obstruction increases, likely because of air trapping (discussed later) [5]. Inspiration is important to measure for many other reasons. One, the variability in FVC may be due to variable inspiration to TLC [6]. Two, the flow pattern of inspiration may point to extrathoracic obstruction (discussed later). Three, in resting or lightly exercising subjects, energy to perform respiratory muscle work is expended only during inspiration. And four, factors governing the distribution of inspired air are responsible for maximizing oxygen transfer from the alveoli to the capillary blood. In a healthy upright subject, inhaled radioactive label xenon during a tidal breath distributes in a butterfly pattern throughout the mid and lower lung zones [7]. In patients with diaphragm weakness, little inspired air reaches the lung base. With diffuse airway disease, the distribution of inspired air becomes irregular (discussed further in Chaps. 3 or 4). Regardless of the etiology, altered distribution of inspired air causes hypoxemia.

As noted earlier, the tethering effect on the small airways increases with inspiration and decreases with expiration. Key to this observation is a basic principle of tube mechanics whereby a tube will collapse when the pressure outside is greater than the pressure inside. In respiratory physiology, it is the relationship between the pressure outside the airway (determined by pleural pressure) and the intra-alveolar pressure (determined by the volume of air in the alveoli and the elastic tension of the airways) that determines alveoli size and thus the degree to which the small airways are tethered. During a quiet (tidal) inspiration, as the diaphragm descends and the thoracic cage expands, pleural pressure becomes more negative, which leads to pressure in the alveoli falling below atmospheric pressure (see Fig. 2.2a). The negative intra-alveolar pressure allows air to enter and distend the alveoli. During a tidal expiration, the depressed diaphragm relaxes, and thorax returns to its starting shape. Pleural pressure becomes less

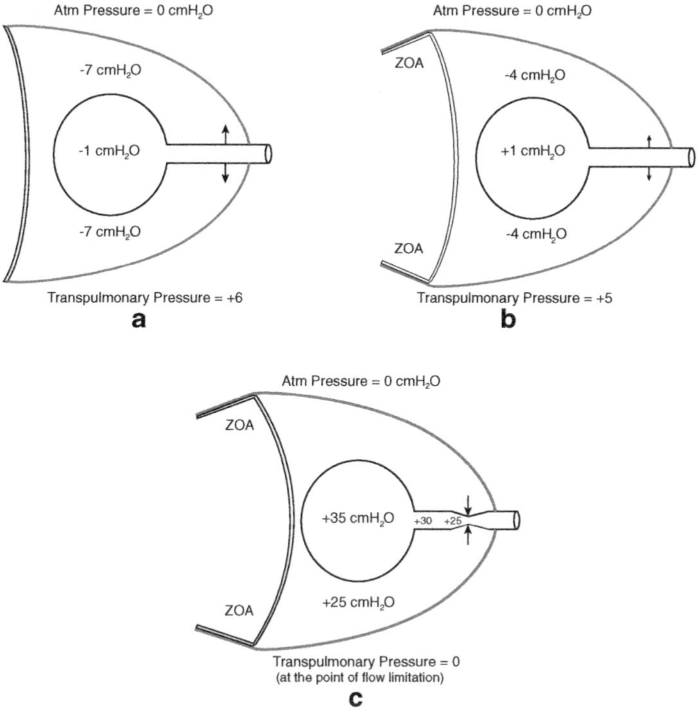

Fig. 2.2 Intrapleural, intra-alveolar, and transpulmonary pressures (**a**) during inspiration, (**b**) during expiration, and (**c**) during a forced expiration. Extrernal perimeter represents the thoracic cavity. Inner, circular area = lung and airways. External minus inner = pleural space. All pressures are in cm H2O. ZOA, zone of apposition

negative and alveolar pressure turns positive (see Fig. 2.2b). As pleural pressure is always negative during quiet respiration, intra-alveolar pressure is always greater, and the alveoli stay open. Thus, so do the small airways.

In contrast to a tidal breath expiration, a forced expiration that follows a full inspiration (as in spirometry testing) incorporates accessory expiratory muscles (see Chap. 7) that compress the thoracic cage and increase both intrathoracic and intra-abdominal pressures. At the initiation of the forced vital capacity maneuver, that is, at TLC, intra-alveolar pressure is greater than pleural pressure because of the elastic forces of the lung (also known as elastic recoil pressure). Expiratory flow rate is proportional to expiratory effort (effort dependent). As lung volume decreases with forced exhalation, both lung recoil and alveolar pressure decrease as well. In diseases with airway muscle contraction and/or small airway inflammation (asthma), loss of alveolar architecture (emphysema) and/or mucus impaction (chronic bronchitis, bronchiectasis) airway resistance is increased. This accelerates the drop in alveolar pressure. The moment at which alveolar or airway pressure equilibrates with pleural pressure is known as the equal pressure point (EPP; Fig. 2.2c) [8]. Because of this EPP, as lung volume diminishes further, maximal flow becomes effort independent. Additional effort serves only to compress the airway distal to the EPP.

To appreciate the equal pressure point concept and its clinical implication, it is helpful to reflect back upon its original description by Mead [9]. The EPP is located within the trachea at the thoracic inlet, that is, the junction between the neck and the pleural cavity. For the physiologist, the EPP represents the transition within the trachea where the intraluminal pressure oscillates with the tidal breathing cycle as thus differs from mouth pressure. The investigators devised a series of catheters that allowed for simultaneous recording of pressures at three sites: one site in the pleural cavity via an esophageal balloon and two sites within the trachea. The investigators, while monitoring pressure from the two tracheal catheters, were able to place one catheter proximal to the thoracic inlet, and, the other, distal, or within the pleural cavity. The subjects were then instructed to perform a forced vital capacity maneuver while breathing through a pneumotachograph. At the initiation of the forced exhalation, the pressures in both airway catheters were identical. At the instant, the peak flow rate appeared on the oscilloscope, the pressure recordings from the two tracheal catheters diverged. The proximal catheter recorded ambient pressure. The distal catheter recorded a pressure identical to the pressure within the pleural space. This study confirmed the notion that the site of flow limitation appears first in the first-generation airway. It also supports the clinical interpretation that the peak flow measurement is a function solely of large airway function. Since in healthy lungs, the FEV1 approaches 80% of the vital capacity, it follows that after 1 second, the lung volume is less than FRC, and the EPP has moved distally, reinforcing that the FEV1 is a measure of global airway function.

Thus in the healthy lung during a forced expiration maneuver, the EPP develops in a first generation airway. As lung volume decreases, the cross-sectional area of airway decreases. The EPP moves distally but remains in an area that still contains cartilage. Thus, there is minimal effect on airway resistance [9]. In patients with severe airway obstruction, the EPP moves peripherally to the small airways, closer to the alveoli [8]. As airways in this region lack cartilage, the pressure differential (outside greater than inside) causes the airway to collapse, a process referred to as dynamic compression. As airway disease increases in severity, an inflection point can be seen on the expiratory limb of the flow volume curve (as seen in Fig. 2.3a), suggesting minimal flow with more air remaining in the alveoli than usual (referred to air trapping). This is especially notable at low lung volumes when there

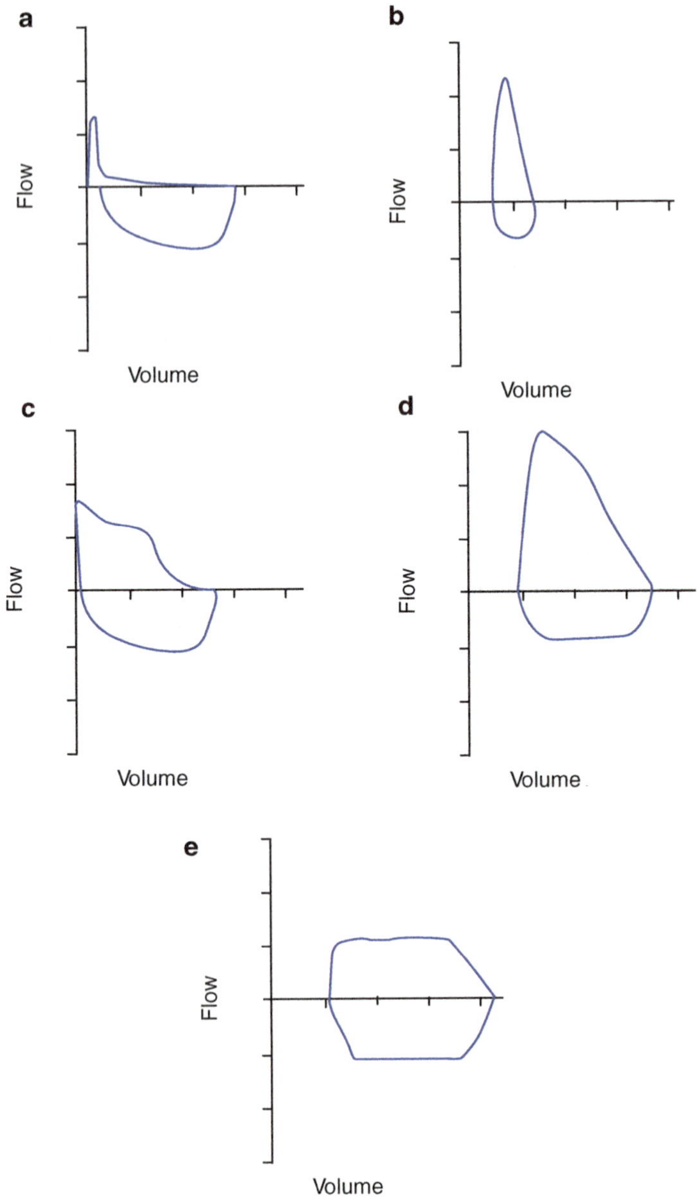

Fig. 2.3 Five flow volume loops obtained from spirometry showing patterns consistent with (**a**) obstruction, (**b**) restriction, (**c**) intrathoracic obstruction, (**d**) extrathoracic obstruction, and (**e**) fixed obstruction

is less elastic recoil. Of note, dynamic compression does not alter the shape of the inspiratory curve because the pressures during inspiration always expand bronchi [10].

Clinical Application

The volume of air that an individual can forcefully expire in 1 second after a full inhalation, the FEV1, is measured during routine spirometry. This value reflects the caliber of both large and small airways, expiratory muscle strength, and the viscoelastic properties of the lung and chest wall. It is reduced in obstructive airway diseases where there is significant airway narrowing and premature airway closure as depicted in Fig. 2.1. When presented as a percentage of predicted, it is used to stratify disease severity of patients with obstructive airway diseases. It has been used to predict outcomes including exacerbation risk and all-cause mortality. The predictive accuracy improves when combined with other clinical measures [11, 12]. The FEV1Q (FEV1Quotient), which standardizes the FEV1 to a "bottom-line" sex-specific limit needed to survive (which is 0.4 L for women and 0.5 L for men) [6] instead of using a percent of predicted normal, appears to be a stronger predictor of mortality [13]. While FEV1 is often reduced in restrictive lung diseases as well, this is primarily due to the reduced lung volume available for exhalation which may be a consequence of parenchymal lung disease, expiratory muscle weakness, or reduced chest wall expansion [6].

Peak expiratory flow rate (PEFR) is another dynamic measurement used to estimate the degree of airway obstruction. It records the maximum speed of expiratory flow, measured in liters per minute. PEFR is less sensitive than the FEV1 [14]. During forced expiration, peak air flow occurs early in the maneuver just as the EPP develops (see Fig. 2.1). Peak flow is thus determined primarily by the caliber of the large central airways [9, 15]. In contrast, during 1 s, lung volume decreases such that the EPP moves distally. Thus, the FEV1 reflects both large and small airways [9]. PEFR is thus not a surrogate for FEV1. In one study of over 6000 individuals with a known obstructive defect, more than half showed a >10% difference between the predicted percent values for PEFR and FEV1 [16]. PEFR is mainly used to monitor response to triggers or medications in patients with known obstructive airway disease, typically asthma.

Maximal voluntary ventilation (MVV) is another measurement of overall ventilatory capacity. Measurement of the MVV requires a sustained respiratory effort with the patient breathing rapidly and deeply over a defined period of time (typically 12 s). This volume is multiplied by five and expressed as ventilatory volume per minute. A normal MVV varies with body size, age, and sex. This measurement is dependent on inspiratory and expiratory breathing effort and may be reduced in patients with obstructive and restrictive lung diseases, respiratory muscle weakness, neuromuscular diseases, or deconditioning. It is thus nonspecific. There is a modest correlation between MVV and respiratory symptoms [17]. In most clinical practices, the FEV1 has replaced this measurement. The MVV is equivalent to the product of the FEV1 in liters times 40. In the analysis of exercise laboratory data, this calculation is often used to compute the ventilatory reserve for a given subject (see Chap. 6).

FEV_1 alone decreases in multiple disease states with different underlying mechanisms. Further, the FEV1 can be in the normal range for a patient who has mild obstructive lung disease. However, when FEV1 is expressed as the proportion of the total forced vital capacity (FEV1/FVC ratio), it becomes an important index to detect airway dysfunction. In a healthy individual, most of the FVC is expired quickly and results in a high FEV1/FVC ratio (see Fig. 2.1). In a patient with small airway inflammation or loss of alveolar architecture, the FEV1 is disproportionately reduced more than the FVC due to dynamic compression of the airways, resulting in a low FEV1/FVC ratio, defined as the fifth percentile of a normal population [6]. To capture FVC accurately, forced exhalation should continue for enough time for the patient to demonstrate a volume plateau such that the value of FVC would not change if the test was stopped, which for some patients with obstructive lung disease, may take greater than 15 seconds [12]. Early cessation can produce a falsely lower FVC (and normalize the ratio) and thus, mask the interpretation of underlying obstruction. Repeated measurements are required to ensure reproducibility with a cutoff of variation equal to when the difference between the largest and next largest measurement is 150 cc or less [18]. In addition, the acceptable FEV1 and FVC values do not need to be from the same maneuver.

While a normal FEV1/FVC ratio due to comparable reductions in both FEV1 and FVC usually suggests a restrictive disease (though requires lung volumes to confirm), obstructive disease is not ruled out. In addition to a falsely lowered FVC due to a short expiratory effort (emphasizing the importance of looking at both loop configurations and absolute values when interpreting lung function studies), the FVC may be only partially reduced in severe airway obstruction due to air trapping, mimicking a restrictive pattern and termed "psuedorestriction." In this situation, the forced expiratory maneuver causes dynamic airway compression, and the FVC reflects incomplete emptying of the airways. A slow vital capacity (SVC) measurement in the same patient would conceivably be greater as this test allows for more complete emptying. A normal ratio in the setting of reduced FEV1 and FVC has also been described in a subset of patients (commonly current or former smokers) who present with typical respiratory symptoms as a patient with spirometrically confirmed COPD, and perhaps even structural lung lesions (e.g., emphysema) on CT scan. These patients are at risk of developing airflow obstruction over time (especially those with a lower FEV1% predicted) [19], and this pattern has been termed "PRISm" (Preserved Ratio Impaired Spirometry).

The maximal mid expiratory flow rate (MMF or FEF 25%–75%) is measured as the slope of the chord drawn from the middle half (between 25% and 75% of the FVC) of the expiratory limb of the volume-time curve. The FEF 25%–75% has been proposed as a marker of patients with obstructive lung disorders. It depends upon an accurate measurement of the FVC, which is not easily reproduced. Further, since changes in FEF 25%–75% are related to changes in FVC, pre- and post-bronchodilator comparisons of MMF are felt to be unhelpful [20]. Overall, the significant intra-subject variability and lack of specificity limit its use [21].

The flow-volume loop graphic in a patient with normal lungs traditionally displays expiration starting on the left, with a steady flow rate upward and then to the right with a steady descent. Inspiration begins where expiration ends and moves downward and to the left in a rounded semi-circle appearance (see Fig. 2.1). Irregularities may suggest some difficulty with testing or pathology. In obstructive lung diseases such as asthma or COPD, the expiratory limb demonstrates reduced flow with a lower initial peak (equivalent to the PEFR) and becomes more and more concave as exhalation approaches low lung volumes (see Fig. 2.1). As the severity of the obstruction increases, the flow is reduced earlier and may demonstrate an inflection point signifying the EPP (see Fig. 2.3a). Restriction may be suggested by an overall compressed loop (see Fig. 2.3b), or a volume-time plot that reaches a plateau early and at low lung volumes (see Fig. 2.1).

Volume-time graphics can demonstrate patient hesitation and inadequate expiration time. The forced expiration should not end until there is <0.025 L change in the last second of testing [18]. Some patients with severe airway obstruction are unable to comply with that instruction. The plot often does not plateau and thus emptying is incomplete. The forced expiratory time may exceed 15 s, suggesting more air remains (and so the FVC will be slightly underestimated). Hyperinflation, or an elevated RV, may be demonstrated by lung volume testing and may provide more accurate assessment offer trapping.

Visual inspection of the flow-volume (FV) curve provides qualitative information that illustrates the nature of airway obstruction. Inspection of the expiratory loop may show diffuse obstruction within the tracheobronchial tree, as discussed above. The terminal end of the expiratory portion of the FV curve of a normal subject will appear to be either straight or slightly convex upward. With disease of peripheral airways, the tracing at the terminal end of the maneuver will appear as concave upward. The expiratory FV curve of an emphysematous patient often shows the formation of a peak flow with an immediate descent to a very low expiratory flow rate. The remainder of the tracing appears as a low flat line. Significant obstruction in the upper airway, in contrast, is demonstrated by a flattening of the entire flow volume loop with the abolition of a peak flow in either the inspiratory or the expiratory limb with lesions above or below the thoracic inlet, respectively. When there is an obstruction anywhere between the larynx and the part of the trachea that is above the thoracic inlet, the pressure differential is between the outside pressure (in this case, atmospheric pressure) and the intraluminal pressure of the airway. During normal inspiration, the pressure in the airways decrease (allowing air to enter), but since atmospheric pressure does not change, there is a slight reduction in luminal diameter. If the lesion is large enough to cause an occluded airway with inspiration, flow will cease and will be demonstrated by a flattening on a portion of the inspiratory limb of the flow volume loop (see Fig. 2.3d). During expiration, however, airway pressure becomes positive and so flow will appear normal. This is termed "variable extrathoracic obstruction" (Fig. 2.4a) and can be seen in patients with vocal cord lesions or tracheal tumors, who often present with stridor. In contrast, lesions in the part of the trachea below the thoracic inlet (and thereby in the thoracic cage) or main bronchi occlude the airway during expiration and not inspiration (variable intrathoracic obstruction, Fig. 2.3c). In this case, the pressure outside the trachea is intrathoracic pressure and is determined by pleural pressure. When the patient with this lesion breathes in, pleural pressure decreases more than intratracheal pressure (inside pressure greater than outside pressure) and so the lumen remains open. However, when the patient exhales forcefully, pleural pressure becomes positive and greater than tracheal pressure causing the compromised airway to be occluded (see Fig. 2.4b). If a tracheal obstruction cannot be displaced by changes in pressure, as in the case of tracheal stenosis where intraluminal fibrotic tissue causes circumferential narrowing, fixed obstruction results with limited flow (flattening) seen during both inspiration and expiration (see Fig. 2.3e).

One final pearl. Rarely the clinician will encounter a test result with and FEV1 of 85% predicted (normal), a FVC of 115% predicted (normal) but an FEV1/FVC ratio of 68% (diminished). This unusual finding most likely represents dysanapsis, the mismatching between airway tree caliber and lung volume in early

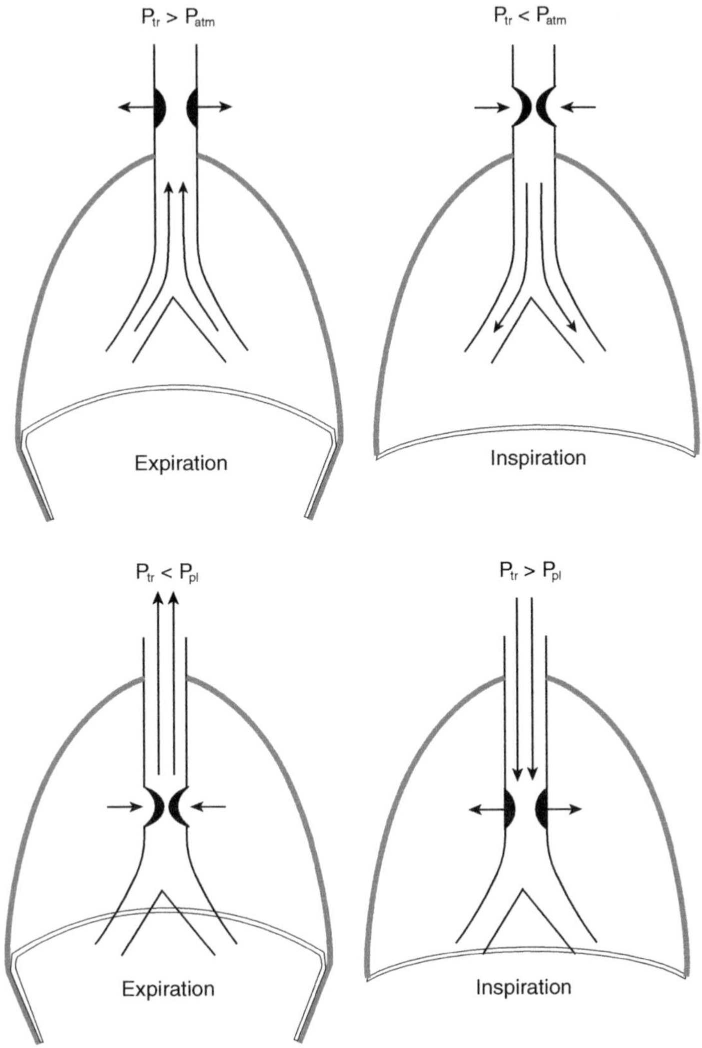

Fig. 2.4 (**a**) Variable extrathoracic obstruction. (**b**) Variable intrathoracic obstruction. Ptr, pressure in the trachea; Patm, atmospheric pressure; Ppl, pleural pressure

lung development [22]. Geneticists speculate as to whether or not dysanapsis predisposes to airway disease in adult life.

Plethysmography

Body plethysmography provides a direct measure of airway resistance (Raw). Resistance (Raw) = pressure (P) / flow (F). The previous chapter described the measurement of an airway (mouth) pressure generated by the subject panting against a closed shutter. That pressure which served to calculate FRC may also serve as the pressure used to compute Raw. The corresponding flow is recorded during the same panting maneuver, this time with the shutter open [23]. The patient is instructed to take rapid, shallow, uniform breaths (panting) with a nose clip in place, hands on his cheeks to prevent cheek expansion and volume change. During this maneuver, the subject oscillates between 30 cc and 50 cc of air at a rate of one-to-two cycles per second. The computed Raw ranges between 1.0 and 2.5 cm H2O/L/s in normals. Resistance is often presented as conductance (the reciprocal of resistance, or Gaw). This conductance is then standardized for the volume at which it is measured. Specific conductance (sGaw) is the product of Gaw and (1/TGV) where thoracic gas volume (TGV) is the volume at which flow is measured. This TGV is essentially FRC [24]. sGaw thereby reflects airway patency independent of lung volume. This is important because in any individual subject, airway resistance and lung volume are inversely related.

The sGaw measure provides a perspective on airway function different from that of the spirometer. To illustrate, maximal expiratory airfow in the emphysema patient is reduced primarily by the collapse of noncartilagenous airways during forced exhalation. In emphysema, FEV1 may be reduced while sGaw is nearly normal. By contrast, sGaw and FEV1 decrease in tandem in asthmatic patients. The sGaw measurement is sensitive for detecting narrowing in both the extrathoracic (upper airway) and the extrathoracic portion of the trachea and in large central intrathoracic (intrathoracic trachea and main bronchi) airways. It is insensitive to identifying peripheral airway narrowing. Thus, it is not commonly used to identify airflow obstruction [6].

Understanding the mechanics of how air flows through the airways in health and disease is essential to understand dynamic lung function testing and its limitations.

References

1. Braun L. Breathing race into the machine. Minneapolis: University of Minnesota Press; 2014.
2. Macklem PT. The physiology of small airways. Am J Respir Crit Care Med. 1998;157:S181–3.
3. West JB, Luks AM. 11th edition of West's respiratory physiology: the essentials. Philadelphia: Wolters Kluwer; 2021.
4. Hogg JC, Paré PD, Hackett TL. The contribution of small airway obstruction to the pathogenesis of chronic obstructive pulmonary disease. Physiol Rev. 2017;97(2):529–52. PMID: 28151425; PMCID: PMC6151481.
5. Chhabra SK. Forced vital capacity, slow vital capacity, or inspiratory vital capacity: which is the best measure of vital capacity? J Asthma. 1998;35(4):361–5. https://doi.org/10.3109/02770909809075669.
6. Stanojevic S, Kaminsky DA, Miller MR, et al. ERS/ATS technical standard on interpretive strategies for routine lung function tests. Eur Respir J. 2022;60(1):2101499. https://doi.org/10.1183/13993003.01499-2021.
7. Ball WC, Stewart PB, Newsham LG, Bates DV. Regional pulmonary function studied with xenon 133. J Clin Invest. 1962;41(3):519–31. https://doi.org/10.1172/JCI104505. PMID: 13864417; PMCID: PMC290945.
8. Voets PJGM, van Helvoort HAC. The role of equal pressure points in understanding pulmonary diseases. Adv Physiol Educ. 2013;37(3):266–7.
9. Mead J, Turner JM, Macklem PT, Little JB. Significance of the relationship between lung recoil and maximum expiratory flow. J Appl Physiol. 1967;22:95–108.
10. West JB, Luks AM. 10th edition of West's pulmonary pathophysiology: the essentials. Philadelphia: Wolters Kluwer; 2021.
11. Wise RA. The value of forced expiratory volume in 1 second decline in the assessment of chronic obstructive pulmonary disease progression. Am J Med. 2006;119(10 Suppl 1):4–11. https://doi.org/10.1016/j.amjmed.2006.08.002.
12. Agusti A, Celli BR, Criner G, et al. Global strategy for prevention, diagnosis and management of COPD: 2025 report. Global Initiative for Chronic Obstructive Lung Disease; 2025.

13. Miller MR, Pedersen OF. New concepts for expressing forced expiratory volume in 1 s arising from survival analysis. Eur Respir J. 2010;35:873–82.
14. Leroyer C, et al. Comparison of serial monitoring of peak expiratory flow and FEV1 in the diagnosis of occupational asthma. Am J Respir Crit Care Med. 1998;158:827–32. https://doi.org/10.1164/ajrccm.158.3.9707093. PubMed: 9731012.
15. Mead J. Problems in interpreting common tests of pulmonary mechanical function. In: Macklem P, Permutt S, editors. The lung in the transition between health and disease. New York: Marcel Dekker; 1979. p. 43–51.
16. Ashutosh N, et al. The relationship between FEV_1 and peak expiratory flow in patients with airways obstruction is poor. Chest. 2006;130(5):1454–61.
17. Ferrari K, Goti P, Misuri G, Amendola M, Rosi E, Grazzini M, Iandelli I, Duranti R, Scano G. Chronic exertional dyspnea and respiratory muscle function in patients with chronic obstructive pulmonary disease. Lung. 1997;175(5):311–9. https://doi.org/10.1007/pl00007577.
18. Graham BL, et al. Standardization of Spirometry 2019 update. An official American Thoracic Society and European Respiratory Society technical statement. Am J Respir Crit Care Med. 2019;200(8):e70–88. https://doi.org/10.1164/rccm.201908-1590ST. PubMed: 31613151.
19. Wan ES. The clinical spectrum of PRISm. Am J Respir Crit Care Med. 2022;206(5):524–5. https://doi.org/10.1164/rccm.202205-0965ED. PMID: 35612910; PMCID: PMC9716910.
20. Boggs PB, Bhat KD, Vekovius WA, Debo MS. The clinical significance of volume-adjusted maximal mid-expiratory flow (Iso-volume FEF25-75%) in assessing airway responsiveness to inhaled bronchodilator in asthmatics. Ann Allergy. 1982;48(3):139–42.
21. Cochrane GM, Prieto F, Clark TJ. Intrasubject variability of maximal expiratory flow volume curve. Thorax. 1977;32(2):171–6. https://doi.org/10.1136/thx.32.2.171. PMID: 867329; PMCID: PMC470560.
22. Yang A, Bon J. Unraveling dysanapsis: genetic insights into airway lung mismatch and COPD. Am J Respir Crit Care Med. 2024;210(12):1391–2.
23. Blonshine S, et al. Optimizing performance of respiratory airflow resistance measurements. Chest. 2008;134(6):1304–9.
24. Stocks J, Godfrey S, Beardsmore C. Plethysmographic measurements of lung volume and airway resistance. Eur Respir J. 2001;17(2):302–12. https://doi.org/10.1183/09031936.01.17203020.

Diffusion

3

Physiologists of the late nineteenth century debated the mechanism of oxygen uptake from the lung into the pulmonary capillaries. Some believed it to be a passive process. Others considered it as a process involving active transport. To test the hypothesis that transfer of oxygen into the pulmonary capillaries is passive, Danish physiologists August and Marie Krogh devised an animal model to study gas transfer from alveolus to capillary blood. Using an instrument—the microtonometer—they had designed, the Kroghs made simultaneous measurement of alveolar and pulmonary venous blood oxygen tension (pO2). They showed that alveolar oxygen tension always exceeded capillary blood oxygen tension. Thus, the process of transfer must be passive.

Next, the Kroghs demonstrated that carbon monoxide (CO), like oxygen, diffuses readily from the alveolus into capillary blood. Unlike O2, however, CO rapidly affixes to hemoglobin. The tension of CO in capillary blood remains zero; there is no CO in capillary blood. CO is thus an ideal marker for the study of gas transfer across the alveolar-capillary membrane. Given this background information, Marie Krogh calculated the rate of gas diffusion from alveoli to the pulmonary blood in man based upon the notion that the rate of this transfer is proportional to concentration of gas in the alveolus [1]. To make this calculation, Krogh needed to obtain serial measurements of alveolar [CO] during a brief breath hold in which the subject had inhaled gas with a known

M. Lavietes, A. Berman, *Pulmonary Physiology for Clinicians*, https://doi.org/10.1007/978-3-032-24303-4_3

[CO]. To achieve this, Krogh assembled a set up that allowed for collection and analysis of [CO] twice, once early again later, both following a breathhold during which the subject has inhaled gas with a known [CO]. This work forms the basis for the single breath diffusion capacity test (DlCO) now in clinical use.

To perform the diffusion capacity test maneuver in a contemporary pulmonary laboratory, the subject sits quietly, breathing through a mouthpiece and pneumotachometer. Tidal breaths are recorded on a monitoring screen. To begin the test, the subject exhales fully to RV. At RV, the technician diverts the source of inspired air from the room to a prepared gas mixture containing two markers: one, an inert gas such as helium [He-i] to be used for volume determination and two, carbon monoxide [CO-i], the gas that will diffuse from the alveolus into the lung. When TLC is reached, the technician coaches the subject to breath hold for 10 s. The technician must ensure that the subject makes no respiratory movements during the breath hold. The subject should perform no Valsalva—or Muller-like movements that may alter pulmonary blood volume. At the 10-s mark, the technician instructs the subject to exhale rapidly. The first 750 mL of expired air are considered to have originated in the upper airways. Given that no gas exchange occurs in the trachea or mainstream bronchi (anatomic dead space), the 750 mL aliquot is discarded. The next 500 mL are considered alveolar gas and are collected for analysis. The final concentrations of the markers, [He-f] and [CO-f], are measured from this aliquot.

The diffusion capacity (DlCO) is computed from the equation developed by Marie Krogh:

$$\mathrm{DlCO}(\mathrm{in\ mL/min/mmHg}) = Va \times 1/(Pb - 47) \times (60/\mathrm{t}) \times \ln([CO - \mathrm{i}]/[CO - \mathrm{f}])$$

Where Va = the volume of gas, presumably TLC, in the lung during breath hold and t = the breath hold time, in seconds. This time is determined precisely from the volume-time trace of the procedure shown on the monitor. Since both markers are diluted during the breath hold by the addition of air in the RV to the inspired gas, corrections must be made for both [He-i] and [CO-i]. For Va, the adjustment is made by multiplying the VC measured from the volume-time trace by the ratio [He-i]/[He-f]. To determine the initial [CO-i], the concentration of the marker in the inhaled gas is multiplied by the inverted fraction used to compute Va.

The term [(1/t) × ln ([CO-i]/[CO-f]] is known as Krogh's constant.

Data obtained from the maneuver appearing on each laboratory report are as follows:

One: diffusion capacity **(DlCO)**, given in mL/min/mmHg or as a percent of a predicted value.

Two: **Va**. While presumably this is TLC, the 10-s breath hold is often insufficient for the compete equilibration of the inert gas label into the RV. The Va calculated in people with moderate to severe COPD then represents the volume of intrathoracic gas that is readily available for the gas exchange process, not the true TLC.

Three: **DlCO/Va**. In theory, a subject with a small TLC and a proportionately small DlCO must have a normal lung. This notion is easily illustrated in the laboratory. A normal subject may perform the DlCO test twice. On the first test, the subject breath holds correctly at full TLC inflation. On the second test, the subject purposely holds his breath at 60% of his actual TLC. The measured DlCO for the second test will be 60% of a predicted value as well. In practice, however, the finding of a low DlCO along with a normal Dl/Va ratio does not reliably identify patients with small but normal lungs or exclude those with lung disease.

In addition, some reports include a fourth datum piece, the DlCO corrected for hemoglobin. In practice, few, if any, laboratories obtain a hemoglobin measurement for use in this correction.

Interpretation and Clinical Application

In order for a molecule of oxygen to reach an organ, three events must occur: O2 must reach the alveolus (distribution of ventilation), it must cross the alveolar-capillary membrane (diffusion), and finally it must be transported from the lung to an internal organ (perfusion). Given that inspired air will redistribute from regions of high to low V/Q during the breath hold, the DlCO measurement does not reflect the property of ventilation. And while it is intuitively obvious that the process of oxygen delivery to tissues must involve diffusion, in truth there are few, if any, clinical circumstances in which the process of diffusion limits oxygen uptake. This notion will be developed further in the next chapter. Therefore, the DlCO test must in some way reflect perfusion. Some look at the DlCO as a measure of the surface area of lung available for gas transfer. Clearly, ventilation and diffusion cannot contribute to oxygenation without pulmonary blood flow.

Conditions in Which DlCO May Be Elevated

An elevated DlCO is often found in many conditions all sharing one common denominator: an increased pulmonary blood volume. These include polycythemia, an elevated pulmonary venous pressure in patients with mild left ventricular failure, and patients with left-to-right intracardiac shunt. Included also are severely obese subjects whose elevated circulating blood volume is accompanied by a proportionately increased pulmonary blood volume [2]. These subjects often have a normal DlCO accompanied by a moderately diminished TLC. Finally, asthmatic patients may have an elevated DlCO. The mechanism here is unclear but may include an increased TLC, a proliferation of blood vessels within chronically inflamed airway tissue, and/or the drawing of blood into the pulmonary vessels by an enhanced negative inspiratory intrapleural pressure in the face of narrowed large airways. The exact mechanism is not clearly defined. Clinically, this is often a helpful point in differentiating asthma from subjects with fixed (emphysematous) airway obstruction, for whom a diminished DlCO reflects a permanent loss of alveolar surface tissue.

Conditions Characterized by a Diminished DCO

These conditions are commonly recognized by clinicians. Diseases associated with loss of lung tissue (emphysema), loss of cross-sectional area of the pulmonary vascular bed (e.g., pulmonary emboli; primary pulmonary hypertension), or anemia are invariably accompanied by a decreased DlCO. Note that both a decreased DlCO and an increased physiological dead space invariably accompany pulmonary embolism. Essentially all diseases of the lung parenchyma are accompanied by a decreased DlCO. The diminished DlCO is often a sensitive marker for the early stages of a pathological process involving the lung parenchyma. Conversely, resolution of the DlCO lags resolution of the disease process and is not a helpful marker to chart clinical improvement. Finally, chronic liver disease is often accompanied by a slightly decreased TLC along with a severely decreased DiCO [3]. The mechanism for this finding is unclear. Clinically this is helpful in that a dyspneic cirrhotic patient with normal chest imaging whose only functional abnormality is a decreased DlCO should require no further pulmonary evaluation.

The notion that a decreased DlCO reflects the loss of the cross-sectional area of the pulmonary vascular bed and thus is a surrogate for the volume of functional lung is helpful in the preoperative evaluation of patients preparing for lobectomy or pneumonectomy. If one could measure a DlCO for each lung lobe, and if the surgeon were planning removal the right upper lobe, and if the measured DlCO of the right upper lobe were zero, the surgeon could predict that the patient's pre- and postoperative FEV1 would be identical. Calculation of a DlCO for each individual lung lobe is not feasible. A preoperative xenon perfusion scan off the lung is however available. If 10% of the label appeared in the RUL, for example, one would predict that the FEV1 would be reduced by 10% by removal of the RUL.

References

1. Krogh M. The diffusion of gases through the lungs of man. J Physiol. 1915;49(4):271–300.
2. Rochester DF, Enson Y. Current concepts on the pathogenesis of the obesity hypoventilation syndrome. Am J Med. 1974;57:402–20.
3. Hourani JM, Bellamy PE, Tashkin DP, et al. Pulmonary dysfunction in advanced liver disease: frequent occurrence of an abnormal diffusing capacity. Am J Med. 1991;90:693–700.

Matching of Ventilation (V/Q) with Perfusion: Arterial Blood Gas (ABG) Analysis

4

The arterial blood gas measurement (ABG) refers to the measurement of the oxygen (PaO2) and carbon dioxide (PaCO2) gas tensions and arterial pH in arterial blood. The measurements are made by the injection of a sample of arterial blood into a gas analyzer. The drawing of an arterial blood sample does not require the same level of technical expertise as do the other measures of pulmonary function. Normal values are as follows: PaO2 = 90 mmHg with an oxygen saturation of hemoglobin approaching 100%; PaCO2 = 40 mmHg; and pH = 7.40. Standard deviations for each value are small. Surrogate measures for gas tensions, for example, oxygen saturation and end-tidal PCO2, do not require arterial blood gas sampling and therefore are used in many clinical settings.

Arterial Oxygen Tension (PaO2)/Oxygenation/Regions of Low V/Q

In humans, both minute ventilation (tidal volume × respiratory rate) and cardiac output (stroke volume × heart rate) vary with age, sex, and height. Grossly speaking, however, ventilation is 6–8 liters/minute (L/min). Cardiac output is 5–6 L/m. Thus, globally V/Q for the entire lung is slightly greater than 1.0. This assumes, of course, that ventilation and perfusion are evenly dis-

M. Lavietes, A. Berman, *Pulmonary Physiology for Clinicians*,
https://doi.org/10.1007/978-3-032-24303-4_4

tributed throughout the lung. This is clearly not true in many disease states. Regions with blood flow but no ventilation, for example, intrapulmonary shunts, are common. These may be seen in lobar pneumonia and with other space-occupying lesions, for example, tumor. Conversely, regions with ventilation but no perfusion occur in the airspaces of lung in which the pulmonary vascular supply has been obstructed, for example, pulmonary emboli. In truth, both the airway resistances in airways distal to the central or conducting airways and the pulmonary vascular resistances in all of their accompanying vessels may vary widely and independently in any diffuse lung disease. Thus in the lungs of patients with pulmonary diseases, a continuum of V/Q relationships is observed among the alveoli.

The *two compartment model* is helpful in that it visualizes the diseased lung as having two clusters of alveoli: one with normal or high V/Q relationships; the other, with alveoli having low V/Q ratios or shunt [1]. This model demonstrates clearly how regions of low V/Q account for hypoxemia in the absence of hypercapnia. The model is depicted in Fig. 4.1 in which tonometers are substituted for clusters of alveoli. In a lung with V/Q = 1 represented by the top tonometer, 50 mL of venous blood mixed with 50 mL of room air produce at equilibration a PaO2 = 103 mmHg. Note that this PaO2 is slightly greater than expected in normals. This is because the human body has a small degree of shunt, presumably intracardiac. Next, consider the two cluster model as depicted in the two tonometers below. Here again, 50 mL of both venous blood and room air are mixed but now in two unequal aliquots: one, representing V/Q > 1; the other, V/Q < 1. After equilibration of gas and blood, the two aliquots of arterialized blood are mixed. The resultant PaO2 = 84 mmHg. This is true because of the unique function of the hemoglobin molecule which is designed to hold large amounts of oxygen in a form such that it does not contribute to the oxygen tension measured in arterial blood.

The multiple inert gas elimination method (*MIGET*) is a technologically complex method for the study of ventilation-to-perfusion inequalities within the lung [2]. While it is a cumbersome process and thus unfit for general use as a clinical diagnostic tool, its investigational use has made an invaluable contribution to our

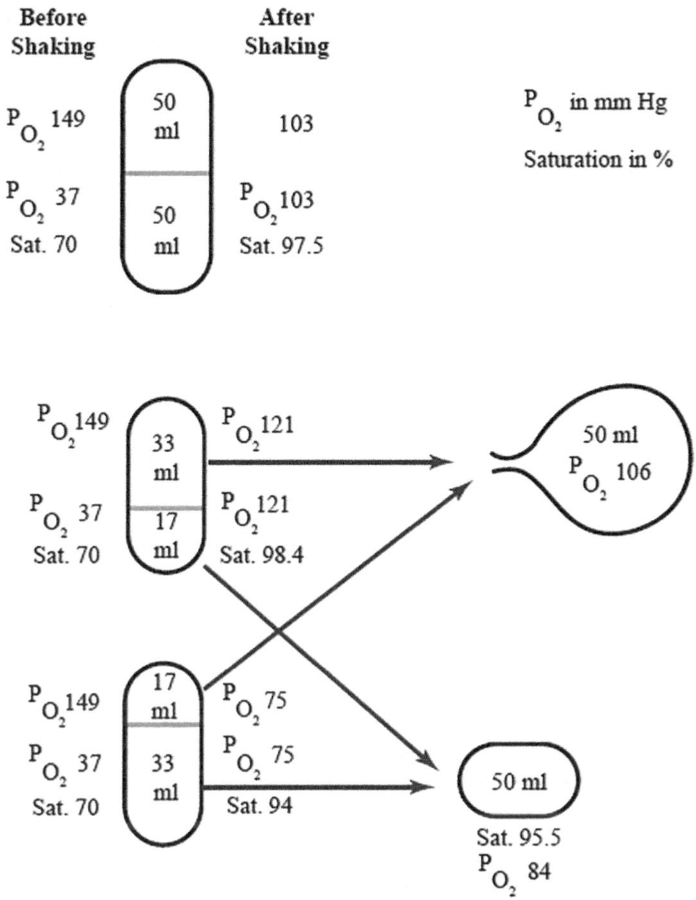

Fig. 4.1 Gas exchange in a single (upper) or two compartment (lower) model of gas exchanging units in the lung. This physiological event is so because of the sigmoidal shape of the oxygen/hemoglobin association curve. (Redrawn from Ref. [1])

understanding of the links between ventilation and perfusion in the lung. While the earlier model considered the lung as having two compartments, MIGET figuratively speaking creates a separate compartment for each of the estimated 100,000 gas exchanging units in the normal human lung. The testing is performed while the subject breathes quietly. The procedure involves the infusion of six inert gasses, each with its own unique solubility constant, followed by the measurement of each of these gasses in the mixed venous and arterial bloods and the expired gas. Processing of these data obtained produces a profile of gas exchanging units unique to each individual subject. The addition of three pieces of information obtained independently, the fraction of inspired oxygen, the cardiac output (obtained from an echocardiogram), and the minute ventilation (from a spirometer), allows for the prediction of an individual's arterial blood gas composition. The plot for any individual obtained via the MIGET process will, in most cases, predict that person's ABG composition accurately. The clinical interpretation of this is as follows: in almost all cases, hypoxemia is explained by either V/Q abnormality or hypoventilation. Note: hypoventilation will be discussed below. The MIGET process assumes that hypoxemia caused by a diffusion abnormality does not exist [3]. In a few cases, the model overestimates the actual value determined directly from arterial blood. The interpretation here is as follows: this discrepancy must be explained by a defect in diffusion. With the use of data obtained from the MIGET procedure, it has been found that a specific diffusion defect to explain hypoxemia occurs rarely. This discrepancy between the calculated and observed PaO2 values is found almost exclusively in patients with interstitial lung disease during exercise.

A tracing from a MIGET study of a normal subject appears in Fig. 4.2. Note that the vertical axis represents both minute ventilation and cardiac output, each in L/min. The horizontal axis represents the range of gas exchanging units from V/Q = 0 to V/Q = infinity. In normals, the range of V/Q units for both variables is limited. Graphically, V and Q curves are superimposed upon one another. The fact that there appears to be slightly greater ventilation than perfusion overall corroborates the statement above; namely, that the minute ventilation measured by spirometry slightly exceeds the cardiac output estimated from an echocardiogram.

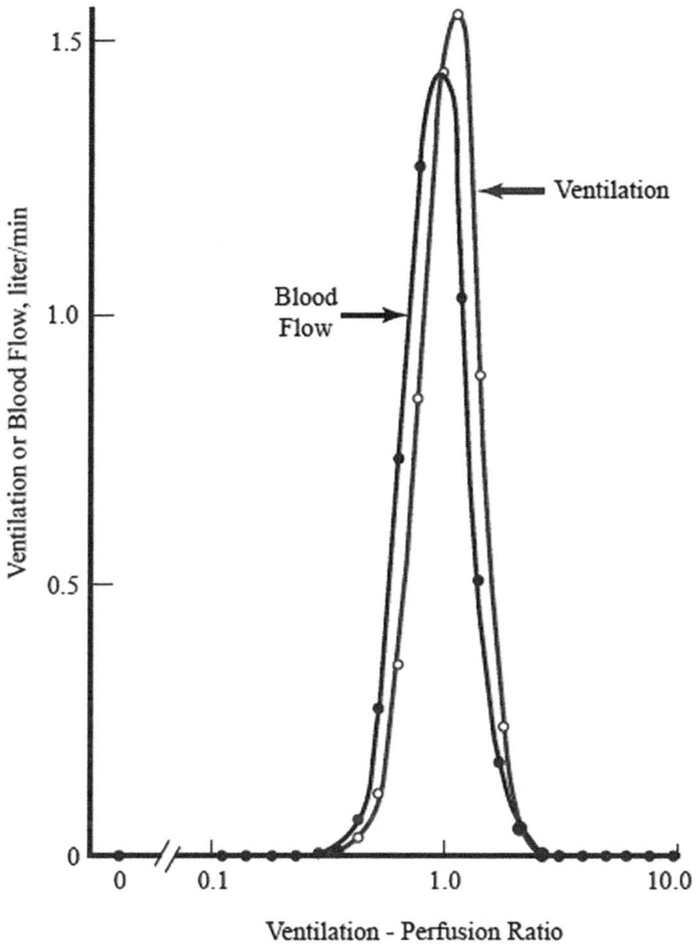

Fig. 4.2 Plot of a MIGET study from a normal subject. (Redrawn from Ref. [2])

A tracing from a MIGET study of a patient with emphysema appears in Fig. 4.3. Note first that there appear to be two curves for both V and Q. Both curves are paired and congruent. The sum of the area under the two ventilation curves appears to be way

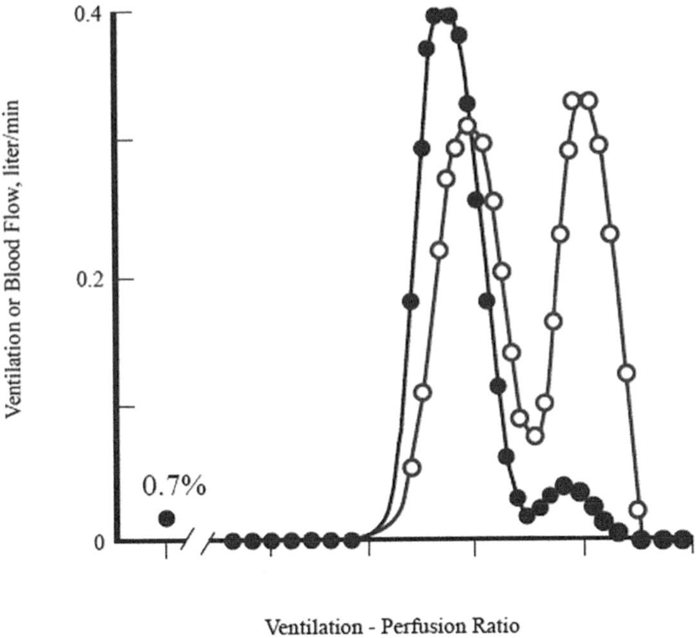

Fig. 4.3 Plot of a MIGET study from a patient with emphysema. The augmented area under the higher range of the distribution curve for ventilation explains the increased physiological dead space measured in the emphysema patient. The label 0.7% refers to the true shunt not shown on the graph. (Redrawn from Ref. [4])

greater than the sum of the area under the two perfusion curves. That is to say, minute ventilation greatly exceeds cardiac output. This goes along with the clinical observation, namely, that the resting ventilation in many emphysema patients may exceed 10 L/min. With exercise, Ve in these patients rises at a rate greater than in normals. This increased ventilation in part accounts for dyspnea on mild exertion, a cardinal complaint of the emphysema patient. [To be complete here, emphysema patients always have an elevated resting FRC. Deeper breaths initiate sensory signals from chest wall/intercostal muscle afferents that are already distended at the end of the tidal breath. This also contributes to the sensation of dyspnea].

Regions of high V/Q, also called physiological dead space, give rise to inefficient elimination of CO2 and thus bring about the increased minute ventilation. We have selected emphysema as our example because it allows us to introduce the concept of the physiological dead space. This concept will be amplified below. Finally, this tracing may imply that the two compartment model describes the distributions of V and Q in all diseases. This is false. In the bronchitic form of chronic airway obstruction, shown in Ref. [4], more blood flow goes to poorly ventilated airspaces. In other cardiopulmonary conditions, more diffuse distributions of both V and Q are seen with no suggestion of two distinct peaks.

A MIGET analysis of V and Q in a patient presenting with acute pulmonary embolism but with otherwise normal lung would elucidate the consequences of pulmonary vascular narrowing or obstruction on gas exchange. Such a study is not available, presumably because this protocol would be both impractical and unethical to execute. Data that simulate this study have been obtained from serial MIGET determinations in an animal model before and immediately following the administration of autologous blood clots into the venous system of dogs [5].

Clinicians recognize that patients with pulmonary emboli are tachypneic. Their tidal volume, respiratory rate, and, therefore, minute ventilation are all elevated. They are hypoxemic and hypocapnic. Their hypoxemia is partially corrected by oxygen administration. Their laboratory evaluation shows a decreased diffusion capacity. These findings are all accounted for by the MIGET analysis. A representative MIGET study appears in Fig. 4.4. Note first the excess ventilation to high V/Q regions. The physiologic dead space for this dog is 49.5%. This accounts for wasted ventilation since little or no gas exchange can occur in high V/Q regions of the lung. Next, note the presence of blood flow to regions of low V/Q. This degree of flow to low V/Q regions is not seen in either normal or emphysematous lungs. The 2.5% shunt (regions with $V/Q < 0.005$) is noted on the graph. This also does not appear in normal lungs. One can think of the development of low V/Q regions in the following way. Excepting the occasional pulmonary

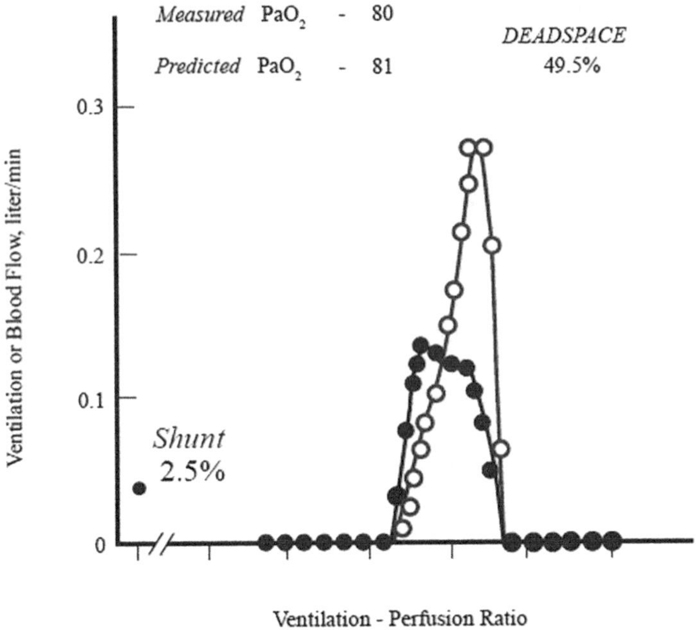

Fig. 4.4 Plot of a MIGET study from a dog, 15 min after the administration of autologous clot into the venous system. The increase in blood flow to both low V/Q and shunt lung regions explains the clinical observation that supplementary oxygen partially corrects hypoxemia in patients with acute pulmonary embolism. This is so because oxygenation cannot occur in shunt regions. (Redrawn from Ref. [5])

embolism patient presenting with profound cardiovascular collapse, the cardiac output in pulmonary embolism patients is normal. The blood however cannot traverse lung regions served by obstructed pulmonary arteries. The normal flow of blood therefore must pass through a reduced cross sectional area of the pulmonary vascular bed. This then creates regions of low V/Q. The clinical observation that hypoxia can be partially corrected by oxygen administration would be expected because oxygen enriched inspired air can reach low V/Q regions but not shunt regions of lung.

Lastly, the diffusion capacity is invariably diminished in the laboratory evaluation of patients with pulmonary emboli. This is so because a portion of the surface area of the alveoli, that is, all alveoli that are normally perfused by vessels distal to the obstruction(s), is bloodless and thus unavailable for gas exchange. The MIGET analysis also demonstrates that arterial hypoxia is explained entirely by the low V/Q ratios in the remaining alveoli. This is so because the PaO2 predicted by the V/Q profile and measured in the subject are identical. The term "diffusion" is somewhat misleading. There is no defect in the membrane separating alveoli from their corresponding capillaries to account for hypoxia in pulmonary embolism.

The *alveolar gas equation* is a simple tool requiring only an arterial pCO2 measurement for computation. It allows computation of the alveolar and therefore the end pulmonary capillary pO2. And from that, the alveolar to arterial (A–a) gradient. This is useful to determine whether the observed PaO2 is a reflection of hypoventilation (hypercapnia) alone or is determined by V/Q abnormality or shunt as well. It reads:

$$PAO2 = (\mathrm{PB} - 47)(FiO2) = PaO2 + \mathrm{PaCO2} / RQ$$

Where PA = partial pressure, alveolar gas, PB = barometric pressure, FiO2 = 0.21, the fraction of inspired O2 breathing room air at sea level, and RQ = respiratory quotient, 0.8 with the average daily diet. Assuming PB = 760 and a normal pCO2 of 40 mmHg, the expected PAO2 = 100 mmHg. While PaO2 may decline slightly with age, for clinical usage, the lower limit of normal is for PaO2 = 90 mmHg. Thus in a patient with a normal lung, the maximum (A–a) gradient = 10 mmHg.

To illustrate the utility of this principle, consider the circumstance presented by many obese people. This is important because the physician is often faced with the task of ruling in or out the diagnosis of asthma or other intrinsic lung diseases in these patients. The abdominal mass affects respiration in two ways. One, it limits the inspired tidal breath from reaching lower or basilar lung fields. At the same time, increased pulmonary blood volume results in an increase of blood flowing through these basilar regions. The result is massive V/Q abnormality from lung apex to base in a patient with an otherwise normal lung. In addition, the abdominal mass requires an increased work of breathing that may result in hypoventilation (hypercapnia). A typical ABG for this subject may read:

$$PaO2 = 75\,\text{mmHg}; \text{PaCO2} = 56\,\text{mmHg}$$

Computation of alveolar O2 here would yield 80 mmHg and therefore an A–a gradient of 5 mmHg (80 − 75 mmHg). This would suggest that obesity alone accounts for this patient's hypoxemia. There is no underlying lung disease. Another simple way to demonstrate this phenomenon is with the obese patient wearing a finger oximeter, ask him to take deep voluntary breaths at his normal respiratory rate. If he has no lung pathology, within 2 min the O2 saturation will increase from its original position, usually in the mid-80s, to 95% or greater. Then, allow the subject to relax. Within 2 min, the O2S will return to its original level. If on the other hand, the patient has underlying asthma, this fluctuation in oxygen tension with voluntary hyperventilation will not occur.

Arterial Carbon Dioxide Tension (PaCO2)/CO2 Elimination/Regions of High V/Q

CO2 elimination unlike O2 uptake is directly proportional to minute ventilation. This is so because CO2 has little affinity for hemoglobin. The efficiency of clearance varies between normals and many patients with pulmonary disease, however. That is so because CO2 elimination can occur only in peripheral airways with no cartilage and little or no muscle tissue. Anatomic dead space then is that portion of the tidal value coming from the conducting airways, for example, trachea and major bronchi. In adults, it is approximately 150 mL. It contributes no CO2 to the airways. Expired air coming from regions with high V/Q ratios also contributes to the calculated physiologic dead space because mixing of air and blood is inefficient in lung regions with high V/Q ratios. These regions of high V/Q have been illustrated above in the MIGET analyses. The term "physiological dead space" then refers to the combined volume of the anatomic dead space and the contributions to the dilution of CO2 in expired gas from high V/Q regions of the lung. The equation governing CO2 elimination, that is alveolar ventilation [Va] reads:

$$Va = \left(0.863\,\dot{V}CO2\right) / \mathrm{PaCO2}$$

Note that Va refers to effective ventilation. It is expressed as:

$$Va = Ve\left(1 - Vd \,/\, Vt\right)$$

Where Ve = minute ventilation, measured directly via spirometer or flowmeter. Vd = dead space.

To calculate the dead space, the dead space equation (dead space/tidal volume) requires a value for mixed expired (me) pCO2. It reads:

$$Vd \,/\, Vt = \left(\mathrm{PaCO2} - \mathrm{PmeCO2}\right) / \mathrm{PaCO2}$$

Where me = mixed expired.

Recognize from the MIGET plot that as regions of high V/Q ventilation such as emphysema appear, CO2 tension in me PCO2 decreases. Physiological Vd/Vt increases accordingly.

Minute ventilation is set by a central regulatory mechanism that may be stimulated by many sensory inputs, for example, metabolic acidosis, pain, fear, and anxiety or diminished by metabolic alkalosis, CNS depressant drugs or severe airway obstruction. This will be considered further in Chap. 5. Respiratory regulation is clinically important also because ventilation sets pH and therefore plays an important role in acid-base balance. Patients with alveolar hypoventilation syndromes compensate for their respiratory acidosis by the renal retention of bicarbonate. This metabolic alkalosis over time blunts respiratory drive. An earlier generation of clinicians treated this condition by administration of oral potassium chloride to minimize the alkalosis. With the advent of continuous positive pressure ventilation, this therapy is now obsolete.

References

1. Briscoe WA, King TKC. Analysis of the disturbance in oxygen transfer in hypoxic lung disease. Am J Med. 1974;57:349–60.
2. West JB. Pulmonary pathophysiology – the essentials. Baltimore: Lippincott Williams & Wilkins; 2008.
3. Wagner PD. The multiple inert gas elimination technique (MIGET). Intensive Care Med. 2008;34(6):994–1001.
4. Wagner PD, Dantzker DR, Dueck R, Clausen JL, West JB. Ventilation perfusion inequality in chronic obstructive pulmonary disease. J Clin Invest. 1977;59(2):203–16.
5. Dantzker DR, Wagner PD, Tornabene VW, Alazraki NP, West JB. Gas exchange after pulmonary thromboembolization in dogs. Circ Res. 1978;42(1):92–103.

Respiratory Regulation

5

In the 1970s, researchers characterized the anatomy and physiology of respiratory regulation in great detail. In clinical practice, however, respiratory regulation is assessed mainly by the determination of arterial CO2 tension. Tension of 40 mmHg indicates normal respiratory regulation or drive. Tension exceeding 45 mmHg (hypercapnia) indicates insufficient drive. CO2 tensions below 35 mmHg (hypocapnia) reflect excessive drive. Hypercapnia (hypoventilation) occurs in patients with severe airway obstruction, muscular weakness, in some patients with chest wall disorders and in patients with metabolic alkalosis or heavy sedation. Hypocapnia (hyperventilation) is often seen either in patients with diffuse lung diseases, with metabolic acidosis or in anxious persons with otherwise normal lungs. Recall from Chap. 4 that patients with acute pulmonary emboli present with hypocapnia. This is not explained by the typical pulmonary embolism V/Q profile. Both hypoxia and afferent input from thoracic sensory receptors may stimulate respiration and thus explain this finding. Also, the notion of insufficient drive needs some clarification. Patients with severe airway obstruction for one example may have normal or increased drive but—because of their lung disease—are still unable to achieve eucapnia. Finally, given the equilibrium between dissolved CO2 with the hydrogen and bicarbonate ions in the blood, pH is regulated by respiration as well as by metabolic processes. Hypoventilation (too much CO2) is associ-

M. Lavietes, A. Berman, *Pulmonary Physiology for Clinicians*,
https://doi.org/10.1007/978-3-032-24303-4_5

ated with acidosis (respiratory acidosis). Hyperventilation occurs with respiratory alkalosis.

Clusters of neuronal cells at the base of the brainstem function together to govern the basic respiratory pattern, that is, tidal volume and respiratory rate. This region of the brainstem is referred to as the medullary respiratory center. When an animal preparation is sectioned cranial to this brainstem region, the animal maintains its respiratory pattern. When sectioned caudal to this center, however, respiration ceases. Anatomically this site is found at the level where cranial nerve X enters the brainstem. When breathing CO2 enriched or hypoxic air, the tidal volume of this preparation increases. Similarly, when an awake person inhales either CO2 enriched or hypoxic air in a laboratory setting, tidal volume and minute ventilation increase. Researchers have assessed the sensitivity of the respiratory center by administering a series of gasses enriched with increasing concentrations CO2 to awake subjects and measuring their resultant minute ventilation. While there is little variation in the resting arterial pCO2 among normal subjects, there is wide variability in their response to inhaled CO2. Subjects with a normal resting arterial pCO2 may respond to inhaled CO2 with incremental increases in minute ventilation ranging from as little as 1 to as many as 8 L of ventilation per minute per millimeter of increased arterial pCO2. Rare subjects with central alveolar hypoventilation do not respond to inhaled CO2. These concepts are reviewed in detail elsewhere [1, 2].

The basic respiratory pattern, that is, the tidal volume and respiratory rate, is set by the medullary respiratory center. It is obvious that input from higher regions of the brain can modify this pattern. Anxious patients, for example, often hyperventilate: that is, that is, to exhibit low PaCO2, high minute ventilation, and respiratory alkalosis. Sedation normalizes this pattern. The rate may be modulated by inhibitory inspiratory vagal reflexes that shorten inspiratory time as well [3]. These afferent reflexes originate from central airways and to a lesser extent from lung tissue and are activated by diseases of those structures. Normal subjects with the onset of stress such as exercise or carbon dioxide inhalation respond by increasing inspiratory flow (inspiratory drive) and thus tidal volume. In many disease states, however, inhalation initiates the inhibitory reflex. When this reflex predominates the increase of inspiratory drive, rapid shallow breathing (tachypnea) occurs.

Note that the sensation of dyspnea arises from multiple physiological and psychological factors and is not related solely to respiratory drive. A recent study demonstrates, for example, that stimulating nasal sensory receptors can reduce the sensation of dyspnea in patients with lung disease while having no effect upon respiratory drive [4].

The use of the occlusion pressure to monitor central respiratory drive has been helpful in clinical investigations but not practical for clinical use [5]. On the other hand, intensive care practitioners use this airway occlusion pressure measurement to monitor intubated patients. Interpretation of this pressure, a measure used to assess the readiness of intubated patients for extubation, requires an understanding of the neural mechanisms governing ventilation. This process has been described in Ref. [6]. To make this measurement, the airway of an intubated patient is occluded at the end of a breath. The subject then seeks his next breath from an occluded airway. Airway pressure is continuously recorded. Repeated trials show that the negative pressure recorded from the occluded airway increases linearly with time and is reproducible at least for the first 0.2 s following the initiation of inspiration against the occlusion. Traces of such repeated measures appear in Fig. 5.1. After 0.3 s, however, the rate of increasing negative pressure is no longer reproducible. It is reasoned that after 0.3 s, the subject becomes aware of the occlusion. His response is governed by his conscious decision either to attempt to overcome the obstruction or to ignore it. Finally, experiments in which normal subjects artificially raise their paCO2 by the inhalation of CO2 enriched air show the relationship between the rise in occlusion pressure with the rise in resting paCO2 to be slightly curvilinear with the rate of change increasing disproportionately to the change in pCO2 with increasing CO2 tensions. A graph of data showing this relationship appears in Fig. 5.2. Taken together, these observations suggest that the measurement of airway pressure 0.1 s after initiation of an inspiratory effort against an occluded airway represents respiratory center output or drive.

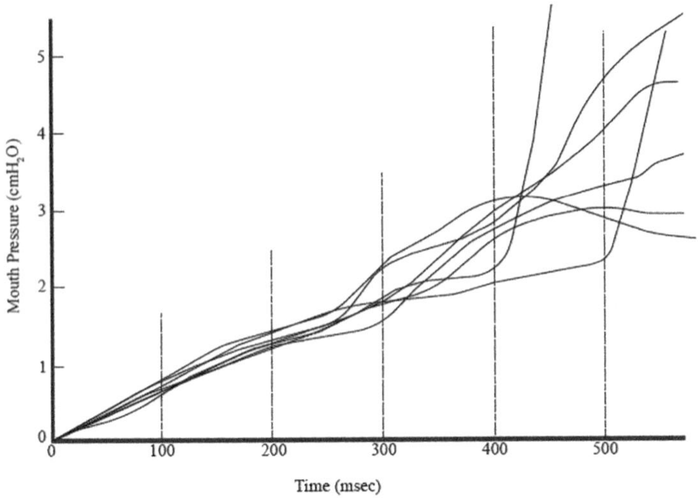

Fig. 5.1 Repeated inspiratory efforts by one person from FRC against a fully occluded airway. Vertical axis shows mouth pressure given as an absolute value; horizontal axis, time. (Illustration redrawn from Ref. [6])

Teleologically, one may think of the p0.1 as a quantitative expression of the brain's perception of the work needed to inhale a tidal breath. Increasing p0.1 values indicate that the brain is anticipating inspiration against heavier inspiratory workloads.

The average occlusion pressure in normal subjects after I second (p0.1) is 1.3 ± 0.8 cmH2O. ICU patients with p0.1 less than 0.5 cmH2O are not sufficiently awake to sustain ventilation without assistance. By contrast, an elevated p0.1 indicates that the inspiratory workload imposed by the diseased lung is burdensome to the patient such that extubation will likely fail. The prognosis for patients with p0.1 exceeding 3.5 cmH2O is poor [7]. Serial p0.1 measurement is helpful in the monitoring of intubated patients. Those with p0.1 greater than 4 cmH2O are likely to fail an extubation trial.

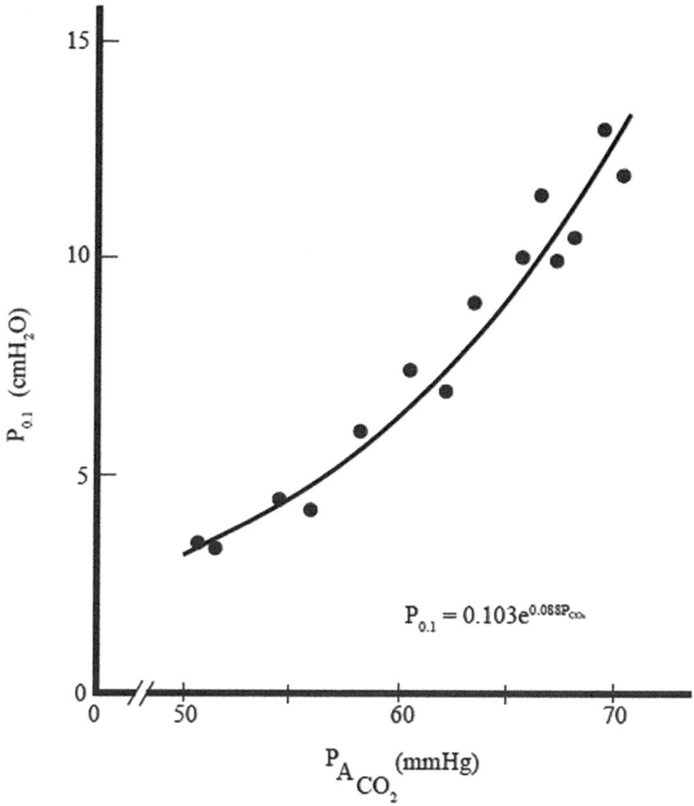

Fig. 5.2 Data from a CO2 stimulation test of one subject. (Illustration redrawn from Ref. [6])

References

1. Hornbein TF. Regulation of breathing, Part 1: Lung biology in health and disease series, vol. 17. 1st ed. Marcel Dekker; 1981.
2. Pokorski M. Respiratory regulation – clinical advances. Dordrecht: Springer; 2012.
3. Trippenbach T, Milic-Emili J. Vagal contribution to the inspiratory "off switch" mechanism. Fed Proc. 1977;36(10):2395–9.

4. LeStang V, Gravwrot M, Kommoun A, Nierat M, Decavele M, Similowski T, et al. Nasal high flow to modulate dyspnea in orally intubated patients. Am J Respir Crit Care Med. 2025;211(4):577–86.
5. Cherniack NS, Lederer DH, Altose MD, Kelsen SG. Occlusion pressure as a technique in evaluating respiratory control. Chest (Suppl). 1976;70:137–41.
6. Whitelaw WA, Derenne JP, Milic-Emili J. Occlusion pressure as a measure of respiratory center output in man. Respir Physiol. 1975;23:181–99.
7. Le Marec J, Hajage D, Deavele M, Schmidt M, Laurent I, Ricard J-D, et al. High airway occlusion pressure is associated with dyspnea and increase mortality in critically ill mechanically ventilated patients. Am J Respir Crit Care Med. 2024;210(2):201–10.

6 Exercise Testing as a Diagnostic Tool

Dyspnea is the most common indication for referral to a diagnostic laboratory for a comprehensive cardiopulmonary exercise test (CPET). For many dyspneic patients, dyspnea is one symptom among a constellation of symptoms and objective clinical findings that taken together suggest a diagnosis. In these patients, basic pulmonary function testing suffices to confirm the diagnosis and quantify the impairment. In others, however, dyspnea is unaccompanied by other clinical findings. Therefore, the diagnosis may be obscure, especially for those patients who present early in the course of their disease. Their condition may not be apparent on basic lung or cardiac function testing. Measurements made during stress, for example, exercise, on the other hand may elicit subtle functional abnormality and suggest a diagnosis. The differential diagnosis for these people is fivefold: cardiac disease, pulmonary disease, skeletal muscle disease, deconditioning, and anxiety. Note that this differential diagnosis assumes a normal hematocrit. Anemia alone may explain dyspnea. The distinction between those conditions associated with organic disease (heart/lung/skeletal muscle) from those without is clinically important. Physicians are often left to tell an anxious or deconditioned patient that his condition has no pathological basis. Patients often do not appreciate hearing this, especially when there is no objective confirmation of this assessment.

The original version of the chapter has been revised. A correction to this chapter can be found at https://doi.org/10.1007/978-3-032-24303-4_8

M. Lavietes, A. Berman, *Pulmonary Physiology for Clinicians*,
https://doi.org/10.1007/978-3-032-24303-4_6

To interpret CPET results, the clinician must be familiar with the physiological basis underlying each variable measured during the test. A list of terms follows:

Variables measuring respiratory function during exercise include the following:

Maximal oxygen uptake ($\dot{V}O_2$ max) Exercise protocols present increasing workloads to the subject, for example, increasing resistance during bicycle pedaling or increasing ramp angle during treadmill running. At lower workloads, there is a linear relation between oxygen uptake and ventilation. At some point in the protocol, at approximately 70% of the subject's MVV in normal subjects, the slope of this relationship changes. MVV continues to rise, while the rate of rise of oxygen consumption flattens (see Fig. 6.1). The inflection point on this graph is known as $\dot{V}O_2$ max. At this point, anaerobic metabolism predominates over oxidative metabolism; ventilation now rises at a higher rate than does oxygen consumption. The physiological basis for this phenomenon is unclear. One proposed explanation is that with increasing workloads, the increasing demands for oxygen by muscles of locomotion must compete with ventilatory muscles for a limited blood supply. Some subjects will stop exercising before this inflection point is reached. In those cases, the peak $\dot{V}O_2$ is recorded. The terms "peak" and "max" are used interchangeably.

Normal: >84% predicted (From Ref. [1])

Maximum voluntary ventilation (MVV) The MVV process has been described in Chap. 2. Given that the MVV exceeds $\dot{V}O_2$ as described above, maximal oxygen consumption, not maximal ventilation, is more appropriate for quantifying exercise capacity or impairment. The degree to which MVV exceeds $\dot{V}O_2$ max is thought to be a measure of respiratory reserve. Note: during the course of CPET testing, other indices of respiratory reserve can be computed from analysis of tracings of airflow and volume, that is, the traditional flow/volume curve. These do not help determine

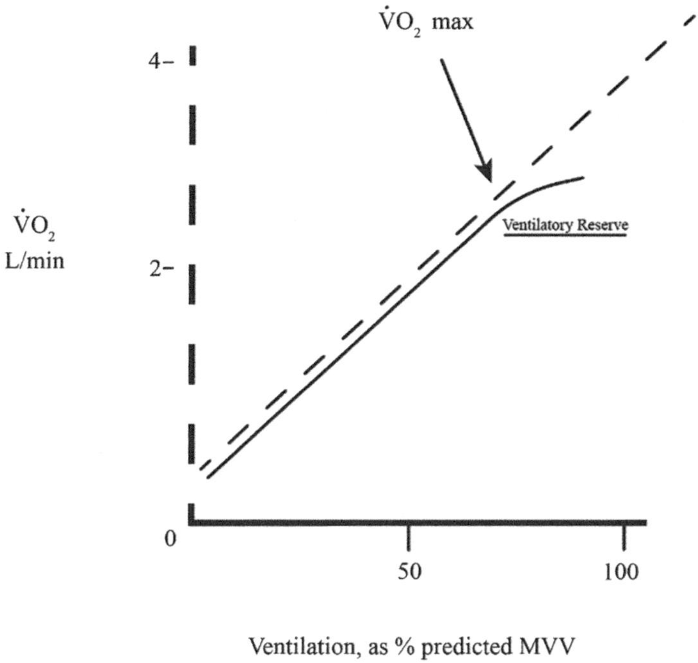

Fig. 6.1 Vertical axis – work rate, given as oxygen consumption / minute; horizontal axis – ventilation. For purposes of interpretation of the test, maximal work is defined as the onset of anaerobic metabolism where the slope of the work / ventilation graph changes

the diagnosis in patients with unexplained dyspnea and, therefore, are not described here.

Ventilatory equivalent for carbon dioxide (Ve/$\dot{V}CO_2$) CO2 production and elimination at rest is determined by the process of aerobic metabolism and is therefore constant. Ve, however, is variable in that subjects with elevated physiological dead space will require greater minute ventilation to excrete the constant volume of CO_2 produced. With exercise, both increase. In patients with lung disease, Ve may increase out of proportion to CO_2 production. The ventilatory equivalent then reflects the quality of matching inspired air with pulmonary capillary blood by the lung.

Normal: <30

Ventilatory reserve (VR) = (1 – [Ve max/measured MVV]) Note that Ve max here is the minute ventilation measured at the moment the subject terminates exercise. MVV is the subject's measured MVV. VR may also be expressed as: *Ve max/measured MVV*.

Normal: 72 ± 15%

Oxygen saturation (O2S); respiratory rate (R); heart rate (HR); spirometry O2S measured noninvasively is a surrogate for arterial pO_2. *End-tidal* pCO_2 as a surrogate for arterial pCO_2. These measures are self-explanatory.

Normal R (at end exercise) < 60 breaths/min
Normal HR (at end exercise) > 90% of an age-predicted value

Variables measuring cardiac function during exercise include the following:

Anaerobic threshold Oxygen consumption at rest is roughly 250 mL/min in man; carbon dioxide production, 200 mL/min. The ratio, the so-called respiratory quotient (R/Q), is 0.8. At some point during the exercise protocol, the slope of the CO_2 production line increases and crosses the oxygen consumption. That point of the graph, the so-called aerobic threshold, represents the moment that the major mechanism for energy production changes

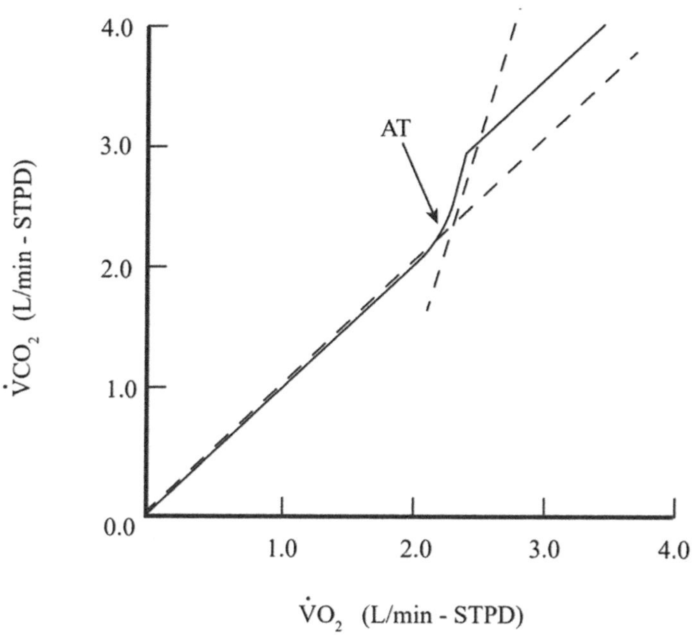

Fig. 6.2 Vertical axis – CO_2 production; horizontal axis – O_2 production. Anaerobic threshold = transition from aerobic to anaerobic metabolism. (Reproduced from Ref. [1])

from aerobic to anaerobic metabolism. A graphic representation of the process appears in Fig. 6.2.

Normal: >40% of $\dot{V}O_2$ max predicted; well-trained persons may have higher values

Heart rate (HRR) reserve: (predicted HR max − HR at end exercise) An overall measure of cardiac health.

Normal: <15 beats/min

O2 pulse ($\dot{V}O_2$/HR) The oxygen pulse is thought of as an index of ventricular contractility. Low slope during exercise suggests inadequacy of ventricular function. The poorly functioning ventricle must adjust to increasing oxygen demand by increasing heart rate rather than stroke volume.

Normal: >80%

Ventilatory equivalent for oxygen (Ve/$\dot{V}O_2$) An increase in the slope of this relationship indicates the transition from aerobic to anaerobic metabolism.

Note: In this presentation, we have included only those variables measured from the monitoring of expired gas. We have omitted many other measures such as blood pressure and arterial blood gasses that require more extensive monitoring. The literature is replete with algorithms and schemes for the monitoring and interpretation of exercise tests [1–3]. The purpose of this text is only to familiarize the reader with the basic principles of exercise test interpretation.

The CPET process involves requiring the subject to exercise with increasing intensity. Continuous measurements of multiple physiological parameters are made throughout the exercise session. There is a myriad of laboratory equipment, protocols, algorithms, and prediction equations available for this process. Laboratories may use either treadmill or bicycle exercise for CPET testing. During trials of treadmill exercise, increasing work requirement is created by increasing treadmill ramp speed or angle. During bicycle trials, increased work is created by continuous adjustment of the resistance required to cycle. The bicycle protocol is preferred for obese subjects because bicycling unlike running does not require excessive muscular work to maintain balance and posture. Because of this phenomenon, maximal oxygen consumption for treadmill exercise is greater than that for bicycle exercise. To be precise, laboratories must use specific standard values for the two methodologies. Laboratories must also choose between gas collection via mask or mouthpiece. There is no obvious difference between measurements made with the two gas collection methods. The mask presents additional dead space to the patient, while the mouthpiece may be associated with some discomfort.

The approach to the interpretation of a CPET test is summarized in Fig. 6.3. Data recorded at the termination of exercise are used for interpretation. Note that the CPET monitor provides a continuous tracing of each variable over time throughout the test. This tracing is helpful in distinguishing the unique variability of the breathing pattern observed in some patients with somatic disorders. Test interpretation usually involves the assessment of the permutations and combinations of the many physiological variables measured in the CPET process for each given subject at the

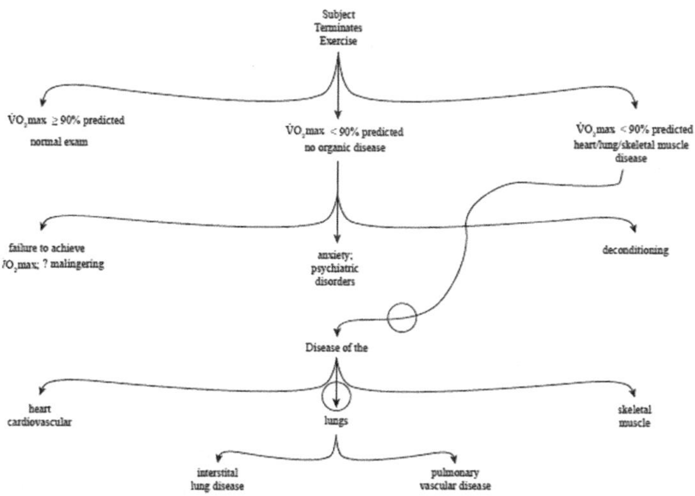

Fig. 6.3 Schematic representation of a simplified algorithm for the interpretation of results from a CPET test. The circles indicate those pathways for which specific diagnoses cannot be made with CPET test data alone and require further testing

termination of the test. Note also that some laboratories report the slope of the relationship between two variables or the slope of one variable versus time as they are measured throughout the test rather than reporting one data point recorded at end exercise.

Interpretation may yield one of three primary outcomes. This initial assessment or interpretation of these primary outcomes based on the $\dot{V}O_2$ max measurement can be made with fair certainty and are thus very helpful to the clinician.

$\dot{V}O_2$ max > 90% of a predicted value Subjects achieving a normal workload may be assured that they have no substantial illness or impairment.

$\dot{V}O_2$ max < 90% of a predicted value; no organic disease Subjects whose data at the termination of their test fall into this category may also be assured that they have no substantial organic disease. Analysis of their test results provides explanation for their experience of dyspnea. One subset of these subjects consists of those who have simply failed to reach their $\dot{V}O_2$ max or are malingering. This group would reach their AT only if they exercised to a workload appropriate for the transition to anaerobic metabolism. Respiratory rate would be low. There would be ample heart rate and ventilatory reserve. A second subset would be those with anxiety or other emotional/psychiatric disorders. They also will reach AT only if they perform to a sufficient exercise level. Both minute ventilation and the ventilatory equivalent for CO2 may be elevated for any given work level. Arterial or end-tidal pCO2 would be low. Note that when an increased minute ventilation is seen in the evaluation of a subject with intrinsic disease, it is usually accompanied by a normal end-tidal pCO2. This is so because in patients with lung disease and an increased physiological dead space, increased ventilation is required to maintain a normal PaCO2. Given that anxious people with normal lungs have normal physiological dead space, hyperventilation in liters per minute brings about hypocapnia. This second subset, anxious persons, may also demonstrate both periods of reduced minute ventilation at some moments during exercise and moments of excessive ventilation at others. That is, they fail to demonstrate the expected linear relationship between increasing work and increasing ventilation. This must in some way be volitional. This can only occur in normal subjects who have failed to approximate or to reach their level of maximal work or ventilation. This is so because as exercise level increases, ventilatory drive increases as well. The desire to inhale intensifies such that at high levels of exercise, that desire cannot be overcome by a person's will to do otherwise. A third subset would be those who are deconditioned. Data from these subjects would show a slightly diminished AT which the subjects invariably reach during exercise. They may exhaust their HRR and reach peak heart rate. By contrast, ventilatory indices will be unremarkable. Note that patients with myopathies will usually have normal indices of gas distribution within in the lung such as the ventilatory equivalent for CO2, physiological dead space, and the arterial oxygen tension or saturation. These people have no airway pathology to account for these abnormalities. They will, however, have other characteristic abnormalities in their CPET profile.

$\dot{V}O_2 < 90\%$ predicted; merits diagnosis with a medical condition While data from the CPET test may be compatible with a given clinical diagnosis, combinations and permutations of the measured variables are such that no combination is sufficiently specific so as to provide a definitive diagnosis of any condition. Only two conditions may be diagnosed with certainty at this stage of CPET testing. One is exercise-induced asthma. Pre- and post spirometry if performed may demonstrate bronchoconstriction. The other is coronary artery disease. Serial cardiograms, if performed, may demonstrate repolarization abnormalities at high exercise loads.

At first glance, it would seem possible to distinguish subjects with cardiovascular disorders from those with pulmonary disorders by means of CPET testing [4]. The anaerobic threshold provides a major diagnostic clue. Early achievement of the AT during a standard exercise protocol is thought to be both characteristic of and specific for patients with cardiovascular disorders. Anaerobic metabolism occurs when skeletal muscle oxygen requirement exceeds oxygen delivery to tissues. This transition occurs early during graded exercise in patients with a weakened ventricular pump. Note that the classification of cardiovascular diseases encompasses a wide range of disorders including ischemic heart disease, pump failure, valvular failure, intracardiac shunt, pericardial disease, and peripheral vascular insufficiency. They share a common denominator: inadequate delivery of oxygen to tissues at high exercise levels in patients with early or preclinical disease. By contrast, the AT is normal in patients with diseases of the lung. It follows that measures of cardiac reserve at the end of exercise would be diminished in subjects with heart disease. Measures of ventilatory reserve would be diminished in those with pulmonary disorders.

The specificity of this analysis, however, is poor [5]. People with occult disease of either heart or lung often show physiological abnormalities characteristics of both conditions during an exercise protocol. There are numerous reasons for this phenomenon. For one, people with any form of airway obstructive disease trap air as their exercise intensity increases. As end expiratory lung volume increases, structures within the thoracic cavity are stretched as well. At some exercise levels, the stretched pericardium can no longer accommodate an increasing venous return. As in restrictive forms of pericarditis, cardiac output in exercising emphysematous patients then fails to match the increasing venous return. Stroke volume is transiently limited. As a result, heart rate increases out of proportion to workload while the oxygen pulse decreases.

At high exercise levels, subtle cardiac abnormalities may also appear in subjects with diffuse disease of the lung parenchyma. With exercise, increasing tidal volume along with the increasing stretching of the diseased lung bring about a transient increase in pulmonary vascular resistance. Granuloma formation within the pulmonary arterioles of sarcoidosis patients may also contribute to increases of pulmonary vascular resistance. Rarely, sarcoid patients present as idiopathic pulmonary hypertension with granuloma formation primarily in pulmonary vessels.

The explanation for a transient increase in airflow resistance within the peripheral airways of exercising heart failure patients is not well established. The notion of cardiac asthma is a well-accepted clinical entity in patients with mild heart failure. The explanation is thought to be edema accumulation in tissues surrounding peripheral airways. The physician would hear wheezes or rales on the physical examination of these patients, however. Thus, these patients would not be likely to present with unexplained dyspnea or to be referred for diagnostic CPET testing. The mechanism for transient airway obstruction is not obvious in patients with subclinical heart failure who may present with unexplained dyspnea, have a negative preliminary workup, and yet experience transitory increases in left atrial pressure with exercise. Transient tissue edema with transient left atrial pressure elevation may occur. An alternate explanation would be based upon a consideration of the anatomical structures of both the peripheral airways and the pulmonary vessels within the lung [6]. At the level of the respiratory bronchioles, the peripheral airways, pulmonary arterioles, and pulmonary venules are encased together within a fibrous sheath. As these structures approach the capillary bed, the tubular structures appear to emerge from the sheath and flow independently into what anatomists describe as a wide cavern or space within the alveoli where gas exchange occurs. Oxygenated blood is then returned via the pulmonary venules. The sheath appears to be nondistensible. The volume of venules increases with increasing pulmonary venous pressure and volume. One may speculate that at the level of the sheath, engorged pulmonary venules encroach upon the space occupied by the accompanying airways thus causing transient airway narrowing.

Given the marked differences between the pathophysiology of the lung in interstitial lung disease and the pathophysiology observed during episodes of pulmonary emboli, one might expect these two conditions to be easily distinguished by physiological measures obtained during exercise. Pulmonary emboli create great imbalance of ventilation with perfusion, creating regions of high V/Q and physiological dead space. Thus, one might expect $Ve/\dot{V}CO_2$ to exceed the predicted value when the pulmonary embolus patient terminates exercise. Lung distensibility in embolism patients is however normal. By contrast, there is little or no airway pathology in the lungs of interstitial lung disease patients. These patients then should terminate exercise well before reaching maximum Ve/$\dot{V}CO_2$. But no measure routinely available during CPET can quantify the mechanical work needed to inflate the lung. Hypothetically, the cycle of intrapleural pressure during a tidal breath can be recorded from an esophageal balloon affixed to a pressure transducer. Pressure recorded during the breathing cycle divided by the tidal volume would provide a measure of work done on the lung during inspiration. While this methodology has often been used in experimental protocols, it is not suitable for routine use in the clinical exercise laboratory.

Given the likeness of physiological impairment in patients with diseases of skeletal muscles, one might expect to identify a subset of CPET outcomes that would be both sensitive and specific to identify people with any or all those diseases. In reality that is not possible. Many myopathies, including myasthenia gravis, Guillain-Barre syndrome, and Duchenne's dystrophy, for example, are accompanied by involvement of the myocardium early in their clinical course. These conditions may be identified by achievement of an AT early in exercise along with abnormalities of the indices of cardiac function at end exercise. By contrast, other myopathies such as ALS or facioscapulohumeral disease may be accompanied by cardiac arrhythmias late in their courses but are rarely accompanied by myocardial failure. Thus, these subjects would terminate exercise with ample heart rate reserve remaining. In practice, few of these patients may come to CPET testing because clues to these diagnoses may be found in routine pulmonary function testing. For example, myopathy patients may have a greatly diminished peak expiratory flow rate with a low normal FEV1 early in their disease course. Given that the peak flow rate is effort dependent, a low peak flow may reflect muscle weakness or malingering as well as airway obstruction. Also, a low MVV along with normal spirometry may indicate myopathy. Clinicians may respond to those findings by bypassing CPET testing and proceeding directly to evaluation for muscular disorders.

Six-minute walk test (6MWT) The 6MWT is a greatly abbreviated exercise test. It is designed not as a diagnostic tool but as a method to evaluate the functional capacity of older people or those with known chronic illnesses and/or physical limitations. It is particularly useful for quantifying the responses to therapeutic interventions in patients with chronic illnesses or physical limitations. To perform the 6MWT, the subject is asked to walk along a corridor for 6 min. Pulse, respiratory rate, and oxygen saturation are recorded before and after the walk. The outcome of the walk is given as the distance (in feet or meters) walked during the 6-min period.

A Case Study A middle-aged individual presents with shortness of breath, unexplained.

Vital signs are normal; body mass index = 21.
Physical examination is unremarkable.
Screening chest X-ray, complete blood count, and cardiogram are unremarkable.
Initial pulmonary function testing showed:

Static volumes:	TLC = 5.07 L (100% predicted)
	FRC = 2.49 L (92% predicted)
	RV = 1.61 L (102% predicted)
Dynamic volumes:	PEFR = 7.1 L/min (78% predicted)
	FVC = 3.44 L (96% predicted)
	FEV1 = 2.39 L (85% predicted)
	FEV1/FVC = 70%
	MVV = 91 L/min (90% predicted)
Diffusion capacity:	DlCO = 16.4 L/min/mmHg (72% predicted)

The patient was the referred for CPET which showed:

$\dot{V}O_2$ max = 0.9 L/min, or 51% of predicted
AT = 0.6 L, or 34% of $\dot{V}O_2$ max
Ventilatory reserve = 0.65
Ve/$\dot{V}CO_2$ at max = 30
Vd/Vt at max = 37
Heart rate reserve = 11 (diminished)
Heart rate = 166 beats/min, or 94% predicted max
Oxygen pulse = 5.0 mL/beat, or 69% of predicted

Summary The reduced maximal oxygen consumption indicates the need for further evaluation of these data. The fact that the heart rate has reached its predicted maximum while the $\dot{V}O_2$ max is half its predicted value rules out anxiety, deconditioning, and malingering as potential diagnoses. The normal peak expiratory flow rate and maximum voluntary ventilation reported in the initial workup rule out the diagnosis of a muscular disorder. Similarly, the normal body mass index confirms the obvious clinical observation that obesity cannot explain this patient's dyspnea. The imbalance between the abnormal parameters of cardiac function, along with the nearly normal parameters of respiratory function, suggests a diagnosis of a cardiac disorder. Further workup of this patient revealed a cardiomyopathy.

References

1. American Thoracic Society; American College of Chest Physicians. ATS/ACCP statement on cardiopulmonary exercise testing. Am J Respir Crit Care Med. 2003;167:211–77.
2. Radtke T, Crook S, Kaltsakas G, et al. ERS statement on standardization of cardiopulmonary exercise testing in chronic lung diseases. Eur Respir Rev. 2019;28:180101. https://doi.org/10.1183/16000617.0101-2018.
3. Hansen JE, Sue DY, Wasserman K. Predicted values for clinical exercise testing. Am Rev Respir Dis. 1984;129:S49–55.
4. Eschenbacher WL, Mangan L. An algorithm for the interpretation of cardiopulmonary exercise tests. Chest. 1990;97(263):7.
5. Neder JA. Cardiopulmonary exercise testing applied to respiratory medicine: myths and facts. Respir Med. 2023;214:107249.
6. Gil J. Morphologic aspects of alveolar microcirculation. Fed Proc. 1978;37:2462–5.

Respiratory Muscle Testing 7

During quiet breathing, the respiratory muscles function in a continuous rhythmic state of activity. The primary muscle of inspiration during quiet breathing in a healthy individual is almost entirely the diaphragm. There are conflicting reports of the role of the external intercostal muscles during quiet breathing, with portions of the muscle demonstrating activity depending on the interspace [1] though their overall contribution to the inspired breath is minimal. When the diaphragm contracts, it flattens and descends by approximately 1–2 cm [2]. It pulls on its insertion points: the xiphoid process of the sternum, the lower ribs, and parts of the lumbar vertebral column, causing the thoracic cavity to expand and increase in volume. This leads to a decrease in intrapleural pressure, and in turn, a decrease in intra-alveolar pressure (below atmospheric pressure) drawing air into the lungs. At the end of inspiration, the diaphragm relaxes passively, thoracic volume decreases, and the lungs recoil back to a resting position, leading to an increase in intra-alveolar pressure favoring air to exit the lungs.

During periods of deep inspiration (e.g., during exercise, laughing, or yawning), the diaphragm descends 6–10 cm [2], the external intercostal muscles contract, and the thorax enlarges to a greater degree. With increased oxygen demand, the accessory muscles, mainly the sternocleidomastoid, scalene, pectoralis, and serratus anterior, pull the rib cage out and lift the sternum and

M. Lavietes, A. Berman, *Pulmonary Physiology for Clinicians*, https://doi.org/10.1007/978-3-032-24303-4_7

clavicles to further increase thoracic volume. This process is known as reverse muscle action because the muscles contract in the reverse direction of their usual activity. Accessory expiratory muscles, including the abdominal, internal intercostal, serratus posterior, and quadratus muscles, move the ribs inward and compress the abdominal wall, thereby increasing intrathoracic pressure and forcing air to move out from the lungs.

Neuromuscular diseases (NMDs) such as myasthenia gravis, amyotrophic lateral sclerosis (ALS), Duchenne muscular dystrophy, and spinal muscular atrophy are diseases of progressive muscle dysfunction that often involve the diaphragm. Thus, they affect both inspiration and expiration. Inspiratory muscle weakness manifests as shortness of breath and hypoventilation, while expiratory muscle weakness is associated with a weak cough, impaired airway clearance, and an increased risk for respiratory tract infections. Unfortunately, and in contrast to most other skeletal muscles, the strength of the diaphragm cannot be directly measured. Transdiaphragmatic pressure (the difference between pleural pressure and abdominal pressure) has been proposed as the gold standard in assessing diaphragm contraction [3]. This test however is not commonly performed in routine clinical practice because the procedure is invasive, involving catheters placed in the esophagus and stomach. It requires subject cooperation and investigator experience. Alternative methods have been developed to assess respiratory muscle strength. These measurements are of particular importance as tests of respiratory muscle strength may decline before the patient reports symptoms [3]. In addition, they are critical to assess progression, response to therapies, or the need for assisted ventilation. Several of the most commonly used tests in clinical practice are reviewed below.

Cough Peak Flow (CPF)

A cough typically occurs after an inspiration which is followed first by a brief closure of the glottis and then a forced rapid expiratory motion. To measure CPF, the patient is instructed to take a deep inhalation and cough forcibly afterward, with the maximal cough flow measured by a pneumotach connected to a mouthpiece. While peak flow meters are commonly used in place of a pneumotach, their reliability decreases when respiratory muscle strength decreases [4]. CPF is often greater than a peak expiratory flow rate because of the higher pressures that build up against the closed glottis. A typical inspiration before coughing is roughly 80–90% of the vital capacity [5] so a reduced CPF may in part be due to diminished inspiratory filling. The expiratory phase of a cough response uses the lower intercostal and abdominal muscles with the minimum volume required for the generation of an effective cough reported to be about 50% of vital capacity [6]. When expiratory muscles are weak, the speed of lung emptying can be markedly impaired, and the force may not be enough to effectively clear the lungs of secretions. A CPF of less than 160 L/min in patients with NMD has been associated with an increased risk of lower respiratory tract infections [7] and is a common indication for an airway clearance device (i.e., a mechanical exsufflator/insufflator). A low CPF, however, is not specific for respiratory muscle weakness. A reduced CPF in patients with NMDs with bulbar involvement may, in part, be due to an inability to achieve a closed glottis and/or difficulty forming an effective seal around the mouthpiece. CPF can also be reduced in patients with obstructive and restrictive lung diseases.

Forced Vital Capacity (FVC)

The FVC measured during routine spirometry is the maximum volume a patient can exhale forcibly starting at total lung capacity (TLC). It is highly reproducible, easily performed, and can be done at the patient's bedside. In patients with severe respiratory muscle weakness, FVC is commonly reduced both during inspiration and expiration. This is due not only to weakness of the respiratory muscles themselves but also to the reduced compliance of the lungs at low lung volumes due to the static elastic load [8]. FVC, however, is a nonspecific marker of respiratory muscle weakness given that it is reduced in the absence of respiratory muscle weakness, as seen in patients with pulmonary fibrosis (reduced lung compliance) or in patients with severe kyphoscoliosis (reduced compliance of the chest wall). FVC is also an insensitive marker in patients with mild weakness due to the curvilinear relationship of FVC with respiratory muscle strength, such that reductions in FVC may not be detected until there is considerable respiratory muscle impairment [9]. FVC is commonly measured in office spirometry and may be a clue to underlying respiratory muscle weakness. Other lung volumes measured during complete pulmonary function testing are less reliable. This includes TLC, which may be normal or only slightly reduced in the presence of an elevated residual volume which can occur in NMD patients in the absence of airway obstruction [3]. Overall, however, the main utility of FVC is as a means to monitor progression of respiratory muscle weakness in patients with known severe dysfunction. While it is used to predict respiratory failure, there are concerns of testing reproducibility at low levels.

Postural Spirometry

Postural spirometry involves the measurement of vital capacity in the sitting (upright) position and again in the supine position. In most healthy individuals, the vital capacity falls 5–10% in the supine position [10, 11]. The positional drop in FVC is attributed to shifting forces on the abdominal contents to exert pressure against the diaphragm [12], to the length of non-diaphragmatic inspiratory muscles becoming less optimal in supine position [13] and to the abdominal muscle contribution becoming more significant. In addition, there is an increase in thoracic blood volume due to gravitational increase of venous return, which increases pulmonary vascular volume and may potentially cause compression of the airways [14]. A fall of more than 15% in the FVC from the sitting to the supine position (representing twice the coefficient of variation in healthy subjects) suggests bilateral diaphragmatic weakness. This fall is significantly related to dyspnea levels, both with a high degree of sensitivity and specificity [15, 16]. In contrast to the patient with bilateral diaphragmatic dysfunction (as seen in patients with NMDs) who typically report dyspnea when supine, patients with unilateral diaphragm weakness are commonly asymptomatic, and have only a modest decrease in FVC, with no cut-off to accurately predict the presence of unilateral diaphragmatic dysfunction [15]. A normal FVC when supine makes it unlikely that there is any clinically significant diaphragmatic weakness [17].

MIP (Maximal (Static) Inspiratory Pressure) and MEP (Maximal (Static) Expiratory Pressure)

MIP (or PImax) and MEP (PEmax) are measures of global respiratory muscle strength. They are performed with the patient seated, wearing a nose clip, and after performing a series of tidal breaths through a mouthpiece. The MIP measurement is sometimes referred to as NIF (negative inspiratory force) though this is a misnomer as force is the pressure over a specified surface area. For the MIP measurement, the patient is instructed to exhale to residual volume and then take a maximal inspiratory effort with the mouthpiece occluded. The recorded negative pressure reflects the strength of the diaphragm as well as other inspiratory muscles. For the MEP measurement, the patient is instructed to inspire to total lung capacity and then exhale forcibly against the occluded mouthpiece, with this pressure measurement used to assess the strength of the abdominal muscles, intercostal muscles, and other expiratory muscles. Both tests are easy to perform at the patient's bedside with handheld units and have become the standard for evaluating respiratory muscle strength in clinical practice. Such devices need to have a small side port to diminish any potential contribution of the cheek muscles. Both pressures are higher in males and lower in older patients, and while normal values are not standardized, a MIP which is more negative than −80 cmH2O and a MEP greater than +80 cmH2O are generally accepted to exclude clinically significant respiratory muscle weakness [18].

MIP is correlated with FVC. It is considered to be more sensitive than postural FVC in patients with mild respiratory muscle weakness [19] and is better correlated with disease progression

[9], though most recommend that the two tests be complementary to one another. A reduced MIP is strongly associated with exertional dyspnea [20] and is associated with survival in patients with NMD [21]. Here again, these measurements can be impacted by other factors and are not specific for respiratory muscle weakness. Patients with skeletal muscle weakness with or without respiratory muscle weakness will have reduced MIP and MEP, though MEP may be preserved in patients with diaphragmatic weakness in the absence of expiratory muscle weakness. Patients with severe obstructive lung disease associated with hyperinflation may have a reduced MIP and MEP not because of respiratory muscle weakness, but rather because of both the mechanical disadvantage of shortened inspiratory fiber length [22] and the effect of intrinsic PEEP [3]. Similarly, patients with severe restrictive lung diseases, such as pulmonary fibrosis, will also have a reduced MIP and MEP because maximal static respiratory pressure is dependent on lung volume. Thus the respiratory muscles of these patients are not at their maximal operating length and thus less efficient in achieving full expansion [23].

SNIP (Sniff Nasal Inspiratory Pressure)

A sniff is a short forceful inspiratory maneuver typically starting at functional residual volume. When measured it serves as another indirect test of inspiratory muscle function, measuring the pressure generated by the diaphragm and other inspiratory muscles. The SNIP test involves asking a patient to sniff quickly, with a catheter-mounted pressure transducer in one nostril while the other nostril is plugged. The pressure recorded has been shown to approximate esophageal pressure [24]. The higher the pressure, the greater the strength of the inspiration. While normal reference ranges have been published, they are most helpful when high, as a SNIP of greater than 70 cmH2O in males and 60 cmH2O in females typically excludes clinically significant inspiratory muscle weakness [3]. Lower values may be confounded by patient effort, device interface, and, in patients with severe COPD, hyperinflation (see above discussion). Some normal subjects can generate higher pressures during the SNIP test versus that measured during a MIP maneuver, perhaps because a sniff involves a rapid, coordinated contraction of the inspiratory muscles while the MIP test involves a sustained isometric contraction. SNIP and MIP are best used as complementary measures of inspiratory muscle strength, and when taken together, increase diagnostic accuracy [25]. The SNIP test is most useful if the sniff is a maximal effort and the patient does not have significant nasal congestion and may be preferred to a MIP in patients with facial weakness. Like the previously discussed tests, SNIP may be reduced in the setting of significant lung disease. In patients with ALS, a markedly reduced SNIP (<35%) is predictive of ventilatory failure [26].

Ultrasound-Guided Testing

With the expanding use of ultrasound as a noninvasive diagnostic tool, clinicians have begun to adopt this modality for bedside assessment of diaphragmatic structure and function. Ultrasonography allows for the real-time visualization of the movement of the dome of the diaphragm during quiet breathing, sniffing and deep breathing, and can reveal diaphragmatic dysfunction or paralysis. This technique, however, does not visualize the muscular component of the diaphragm and may be inaccurate. A recent systematic review showed a weak-to-moderate correlation of diaphragmatic excursion with MIP and SNIP [27]. Contraction velocity, the diaphragmatic excursion divided by the time spent in inspiration, has been proposed as a key indicator of diaphragmatic function, though more studies are needed. Lastly, diaphragm thickness, measured in the zone of apposition (the area where the diaphragm abuts the lower rib cage, see Fig. 7.1) on expiration and compared with deep inspiration, is another tool used to assess diaphragmatic function. While the diaphragm in a healthy individual thickens as it shortens during inspiration, a diaphragm that does not thicken during inspiration is diagnostic of diaphragmatic paralysis [28]. The absence of thickening on inspiration is indicative of the absence of shortening and is associated with diminished muscle strength [29]. This test can be used to

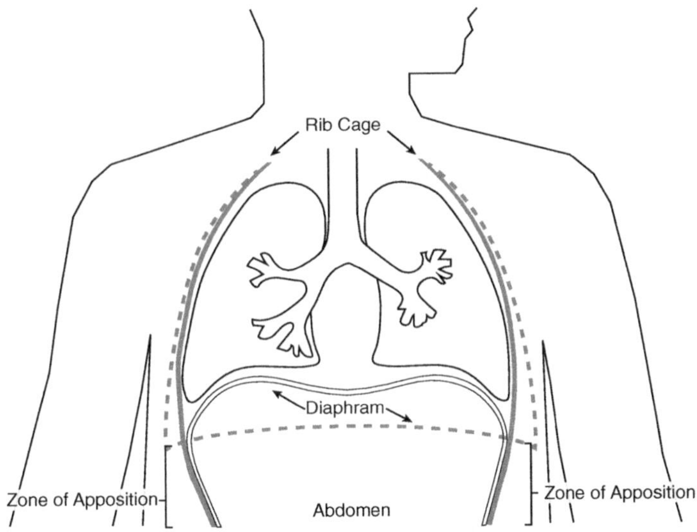

Fig. 7.1 At inspiration (solid line), the diaphragm is a dome-shaped muscle extending over the abdomen. During deep inspiration (dotted line), the diaphragm contracts (flattens) as do the external intercostal muscles which causes the outward and upward movement of the ribs, and the volume of the thoracic cage to increase. The zone of apposition is the lateral portion of the lower thorax where the muscle fibers of the costal diaphragm insert into the rib cage

evaluate unilateral and bilateral diaphragm paralysis. Ultrasonography of the diaphragm has also been proposed as a tool to assess the ability to liberate a patient from a ventilator.

Respiratory muscle weakness is an important diagnosis. Treatment exists for many of the etiologies, and are more effective if administered early in the disease. Tests for respiratory muscle strength are helpful in monitoring progression and are useful in deciding the time to initiate ventilatory support and airway clearance devices. Currently, most patients can be evaluated noninvasively and at the bedside by measuring FVC, MIP, and MEP and incorporating ultrasonography.

A final note about the area of apposition. Recall the earlier discussion of the link between abdominal pressure and lung volumes. Increased abdominal pressure brings about both increased rib cage volume and decreased thoracic gas volume at end expiration. The area of apposition is the vehicle for these changes.

References

1. De Troyer A, Kirkwood PA, Wilson TA. Respiratory action of the intercostal muscles. Physiol Rev. 2005;85(2):717–56.
2. Boussuges A, Gole Y, Blanc P. Diaphragmatic motion studied by m-mode ultrasonography: methods, reproducibility, and normal values. Chest. 2009;135(2):391–400. https://doi.org/10.1378/chest.08-1541. Epub 2008 Nov 18. PMID: 19017880.
3. American Thoracic Society/European Respiratory Society. ATS/ERS Statement on respiratory muscle testing. Am J Respir Crit Care Med. 2002;166(4):518–624. https://doi.org/10.1164/rccm.166.4.518.
4. Sancho J, Servera E, Díaz J, Marín J. Comparison of peak cough flows measured by pneumotachograph and a portable peak flow meter. Am J Phys Med Rehabil. 2004;83(8):608–12. https://doi.org/10.1097/01.phm.0000133431.70907.a2. PMID: 15277962.
5. Mellies U, Goebel C. Optimum insufflation capacity and peak cough flow in neuromuscular disorders. Ann Am Thorac Soc. 2014;11(10):1560–8.
6. Brennan M, McDonnell MJ, et al. The use of cough peak flow in the assessment of respiratory function in clinical practice – a narrative review. Respir Med. 2022;193:106740.
7. Bach JR, Ishikawa Y, Kim H. Prevention of pulmonary morbidity for patients with Duchenne muscular dystrophy. Chest. 1997;112(4):1024–8.
8. Patel N, Chong K, Baydur A. Methods and applications in respiratory physiology: respiratory mechanics, drive and muscle function in neuromuscular and chest wall disorders. Front Physiol. 2022;13:838414. https://doi.org/10.3389/fphys.2022.838414. PMID: 35774289; PMCID: PMC9237333.
9. DeTroyer A. Analysis of lung volume restriction in patients with respiratory muscle weakness. Thorax. 1980;35:603–10.
10. Black LF, Hyatt RE. Maximal respiratory pressures: normal values and relationship to age and sex. Am Rev Respir Dis. 1969;99:696–702.
11. Allen SM, Hunt B, Green M. Fall in vital capacity with posture. Br J Dis Chest. 1985;79(3):267–71. PMID: 4015957.
12. Lechtzin N, Wiener CM, Shade DM, Clawson L, Diette GB. Spirometry in the supine position improves the detection of diaphragmatic weakness in patients with amyotrophic lateral sclerosis. Chest. 2002;121(2):436–42. https://doi.org/10.1378/chest.121.2.436. PMID: 11834654.

13. Segizbaeva MO, Pogodin MA, Aleksandrova NP. Effects of body positions on respiratory muscle activation during maximal inspiratory maneuvers. Adv Exp Med Biol. 2013;756:355–63.
14. Chase SC, Taylor BJ, Cross TJ, Coffman KE, Olson LJ, Johnson BD. Influence of thoracic fluid compartments on pulmonary congestion in chronic heart failure. J Card Fail. 2017;23(9):690–6. https://doi.org/10.1016/j.cardfail.2017.07.394. PMCID: PMC5585067; NIHMSID: NIHMS898730; PMID: 28716688.
15. Brault M, Gabrysz-Forget F, Dubé B-P. Predictive value of positional change in vital capacity to identify diaphragm dysfunction. Adv Exp Med Biol. 2013;756:355–63.
16. Allen SM, Hunt B, Green M. Fall in vital capacity with posture. Br J Dis Chest. 1985;79:267–71. https://doi.org/10.1016/0007-0971(85)90047-6.
17. Mier-Jedrzejowicz A, Brophy C, Moxham J, Green M. Assessment of diaphragm weakness. Am Rev Respir Dis. 1988;137:877–83.
18. Laveneziana P, Albuquerque A, Aliverti A. ERS statement on respiratory muscle testing at rest and during exercise. Eur Respir J. 2019;53(6):1801214. https://doi.org/10.1183/13993003.01214-2018.
19. Black LF, Hyatt RE. Maximal static respiratory pressures in generalised neuromuscular disease. Am Rev Respir Dis. 1971;103:641–50.
20. Killian KJ, Jones NL. Respiratory muscles and dyspnea. Clin Chest Med. 1988;9:237–48.
21. Schoser B, Fong E, Geberhiwot T, Hughes D, Kissel JT, Madathil SC, Orlikowski D, Polkey MI, Roberts M, Tiddens HA, Young P. Maximum inspiratory pressure as a clinically meaningful trial endpoint for neuromuscular diseases: a comprehensive review of the literature. Orphanet J Rare Dis. 2017;12(1):52. https://doi.org/10.1186/s13023-017-0598-0. PMID: 28302142; PMCID: PMC5353799.
22. Polkey MI. Diaphragm strength in chronic obstructive pulmonary disease. Am J Respir Crit Care Med. 1996;154(5):1310–7.
23. Rochester DF. Tests of respiratory muscle function. Clin Chest Med. 1988;9:249–61.
24. Heritie. Sniff nasal pressure: a non-invasive assessment of inspiratory muscle strength. Am J Respir Crit Care Med. 1994;150:1678–83.
25. Steier J, Kaul S, Seymour J, Jolley C, Rafferty G, Man W, Luo YM, Roughton M, Polkey MI, Moxham J. The value of multiple tests of respiratory muscle strength. Thorax. 2007;62(11):975–80. https://doi.org/10.1136/thx.2006.072884. Epub2007 Jun 8. PMID: 17557772; PMCID: PMC2117126.
26. Morgan RK, McNally S, Alexander M, Conroy R, Hardiman O, Costello RW. Use of Sniff nasal-inspiratory force to predict survival in amyotrophic lateral sclerosis. Am J Respir Crit Care Med. 2005;171(3):269–74. https://doi.org/10.1164/rccm.200403-314oc.
27. Leote J, Monteiro M, Rocha C, Rodrigues C, Pereira M, Luz Antunes M, Dias H. Diaphragm ultrasound for muscle strength assessment: a system-

atic literature review. Pulmonology. 2025;31(1):2572252. https://doi.org/10.1080/25310429.2025.2572252.
28. McCool FD, Tzelepis GE. Dysfunction of the diaphragm. N Engl J Med. 2012;366:932–42.
29. Gottesman E, McCool FD. Ultrasound evaluation of the paralyzed diaphragm. Am J Respir Crit Care Med. 1997;155:1570–4.

Correction to: Exercise Testing as a Diagnostic Tool

Correction to:
Chapter 6 in: M. Lavietes, A. Berman, *Pulmonary Physiology for Clinicians*, https://doi.org/10.1007/978-3-032-24303-4_6

The chapter was inadvertently published with incorrect values, where oxygen consumption at rest was stated as 200 mL/min and carbon dioxide production as 250 mL/min. This has now been corrected to 250 mL/min for oxygen consumption and 200 mL/min for carbon dioxide production.

The updated version of this chapter can be found at
https://doi.org/10.1007/978-3-032-24303-4_6

M. Lavietes, A. Berman, *Pulmonary Physiology for Clinicians*,
https://doi.org/10.1007/978-3-032-24303-4_8

Index

A
Afferent reflexes, 54
Airway pressure, 55
Alveolar gas equation, 49
Alveolar hypoventilation syndromes, 51
Anaerobic threshold, 62
Anatomic dead space, 50, 51
Arterial blood gas measurement (ABG), 41
Arterial carbon dioxide tension (PaCO2), 50–51
Arterial oxygen tension (PaO2), 41–50
Asthma, 18, 22, 26
Atmospheric pressure, 20, 29, 30

B
Body plethysmography, 31
Bronchiectasis, 18, 22

C
Carbon monoxide (CO), 35–37
Cardiac asthma, 69
Chest wall, 9–12, 14, 15
Chronic bronchitis, 22
Clinical pulmonary function test, 1
CO2 elimination, 50–51
CO2 stimulation test, 57
Comprehensive cardiopulmonary exercise test (CPET), 59, 60, 64, 65, 67, 69–71
Cough peak flow (CPF), 74–75

D
Diaphragm, 73, 74, 76–80
Diffusion capacity (DlCO), 5
- CO, 35, 36
- decreased, 39
- gas exchange process, 37
- increased pulmonary blood volume, 38
- interpretation and clinical application, 37–38
- Krogh's constant, 37
- passive process, 35
- resolution, 39

Distribution of ventilation, 37
Dynamic compression, 23, 25, 26
Dyspnea, 59, 66, 72

M. Lavietes, A. Berman, *Pulmonary Physiology for Clinicians*,
https://doi.org/10.1007/978-3-032-24303-4

E
Elastic recoil pressure, 22
Emphysema, 18, 22, 27, 31
Equal pressure point (EPP), 22, 23, 25
Eucapnia, 53
Expiratory reserve volume (ERV), 2, 10
Extrathoracic airways, 18

F
FEV1Quotient (FEV1Q), 25
Flow-volume (FV) curve, 28
Forced expiratory volume in one second (FEV1), 19, 23, 25–27, 29, 31
Forced vital capacity (FVC), 19, 20, 26, 27, 29, 75–77, 80
Functional residual capacity (FRC), 1–6, 9, 10, 12–15

G
Gas exchange process, 37
Gas transfer, 35, 38

H
Heart rate (HR), 62–64
Heart rate reserve (HRR), 63, 67
Hypercapnia, 42, 49, 50, 53
Hyperventilation, 53
Hypocapnia, 53
Hypoventilation, 53, 54
Hypoxemia, 42, 44, 47, 48, 50

I
Intra-alveolar pressure, 20–22
Intrapleural pressure, 21
Intrathoracic airways, 17–19
Intrathoracic pressure, 29
Intratracheal pressure, 29

K
Krogh's constant, 37

L
Law of LaPlace, 18
Lobectomy, 39
Lung clearance index (LCI), 4
Lung function, 2, 9, 10
Lung parenchyma, 39

M
Matching of ventilation (V/Q), 41, 42, 44, 47, 50, 51
Maximal expiratory pressure (MEP), 77–78, 80
Maximal inspiratory pressure (MIP), 77–80
Maximal mid expiratory flow rate (MMF), 27
Maximal oxygen uptake (VO2 max), 60
Maximum voluntary ventilation (MVV), 26, 60, 62, 70, 71
Medullary respiratory center, 54
Microtonometer, 35
Mucus impaction, 22
Multiple inert gas elimination method (MIGET), 42–49, 51

N
N2 washout method, 2
Neuromuscular diseases (NMDs), 74

O
Obstructive ventilatory defect
  anatomy and physiology, 17–25
  clinical application, 25–31
  plethysmography, 31–32
Occlusion pressure, 55, 56

Oxygenation, 41–50
Oxygen saturation (O2S), 62

P

Peak expiratory flow rate (PEFR), 25, 26
PEmax, *see* Maximal expiratory pressure
Physiological dead space, 46, 47, 51
PImax, *see* Maximal inspiratory pressure
Plethysmography, 5, 31–32
Pleural pressure, 20–22, 29, 30
Pneumonectomy, 39
Poiseuille's Law, 18
Positive end expiratory pressure (PEEP), 12, 15
Postural spirometry, 76, 77
Preserved Ratio Impaired Spirometry (PRISm), 27
Psuedorestriction, 27
Pulmonary emboli, 69
Pulmonary venous blood oxygen tension (pO2), 35

R

Reciprocal of resistance (Gaw), 31
Regions of high V/Q, 50–51
Regions of low V/Q, 41–50
Residual volume (RV), 1–3, 5, 8–10
Respiratory muscle testing
- cough peak flow, 74–75
- FVC, 75
- MIP/MEP, 77–78
- postural spirometry, 76, 77
- SNIP, 78–79
- ultrasound-guided testing, 79–81

Respiratory muscle weakness, 80
Respiratory physiology, 20
Respiratory rate (R), 62
Respiratory regulation, 54–57
Respiratory system recoil pressure, 15
Restrictive ventilatory defect
- differential diagnosis, 9–10
- physiology, 10–15
- respiratory system recoil pressure, 15

Roentgenographic methods, 2

S

Sensation of dyspnea, 55
Silent zone, 19
Six-minute walk test (6MWT), 71
Sniff nasal inspiratory pressure (SNIP), 78–79
Specific conductance (sGaw), 31
Spirometry, 1, 62, 67, 70
Subsegmental bronchi, 19

T

Tachypnea, 55
Total lung capacity (TLC), 1–3, 5–10, 12, 19, 22, 75, 76
Transpulmonary pressure, 21
Tube mechanics, 20
Two compartment model, 42, 47

U

Ultrasonography, 79, 80
Ultrasound-guided testing, 79–81
Unexplained dyspnea, 61, 69, 71

V

Variable extrathoracic obstruction, 29, 30
Variable intrathoracic obstruction, 29, 30

Ventilatory equivalent for carbon dioxide (Ve/VCO2), 61
Ventilatory equivalent for oxygen (Ve/VO2), 64
Vital capacity (VC), 1–3, 8, 9
Volume of gas, 1, 3
Volume/pressure (V/P) diagram, 10–14

W

World War Two (WW2), 1, 2

GPSR Compliance

The European Union's (EU) General Product Safety Regulation (GPSR) is a set of rules that requires consumer products to be safe and our obligations to ensure this.

If you have any concerns about our products, you can contact us on ProductSafety@springernature.com

In case Publisher is established outside the EU, the EU authorized representative is:

Springer Nature Customer Service Center GmbH
Europaplatz 3
69115 Heidelberg, Germany

Batch number: 10517678

Printed by Printforce, the Netherlands